detox

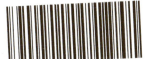

Written by Richard Johnson

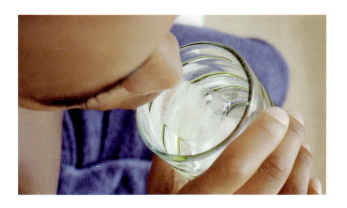

TOP THAT!™

Copyright © 2005 Top That! Publishing Inc
25031 W. Avenue Stanford
Suite #60, Valencia
CA 91355
All rights reserved
www.topthatpublishing.com

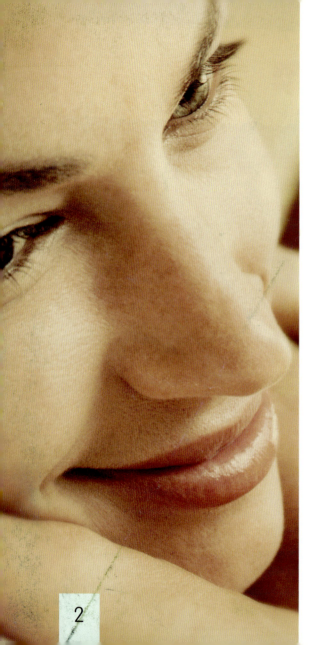

contents

Introduction to detox	4
Why detox?	6
Are you in need of a detox?	10
Body works	12
Safety tips	18
Coping with side effects	22
Detox and diets	25
Planning your detox	26
Food and nutrition	28
Foods to eat	34
Food to avoid	36
Natural supplements	39
Water	42
Water treatments	44
Herbal teas	48
Juices	52
Detox recipes	58

Exercise	**66**
Walking and stretching	**68**
Yoga	**70**
T'ai chi	**72**
Acupressure	**74**
Reiki	**76**
Reflexology	**78**
Massage	**80**
Aromatherapy	**84**
Face masks	**88**
Eye masks and coolers	**92**
Skin brushing	**94**
Body cleansing	**96**
Detox your mind	**100**
Breathing	**104**
Stress reducing tips	**108**
Sleep	**114**
Health spa treatments	**120**
Daily detox	**122**
Glossary	**126**

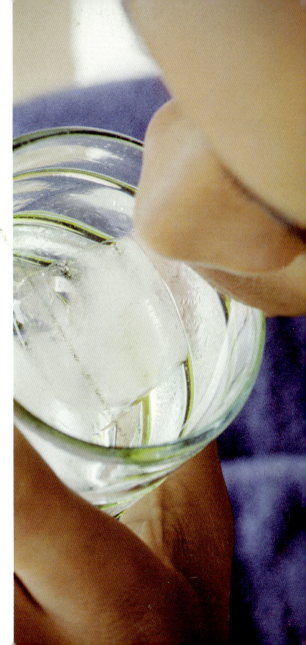

introduction to
detox

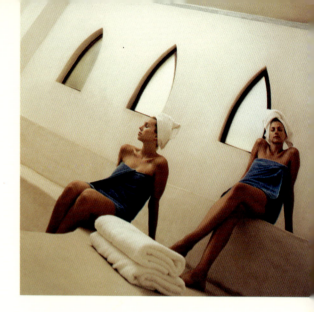

Chemicals in our food, exhaust emissions, bacteria, and viruses are contaminants that our bodies have to cope with on a daily basis. Have you ever wondered how they affect us? Do you ever wake up in the morning still feeling tired and drowsy? Do you lack energy? Is your memory poor? Does your skin look grey and dull? Do you have constant colds, infections and a poor level of general health?

These are just some of the effects that pollutants have on our bodies. The majority of us would dismiss these symptoms and carry on suffering, using stimulants such as caffeine and nicotine to get us through the day. How can we deal with these pollutants when we are bombarded with them daily? The answer is really quite simple: an effective cleansing of our bodies, in other words, detox!

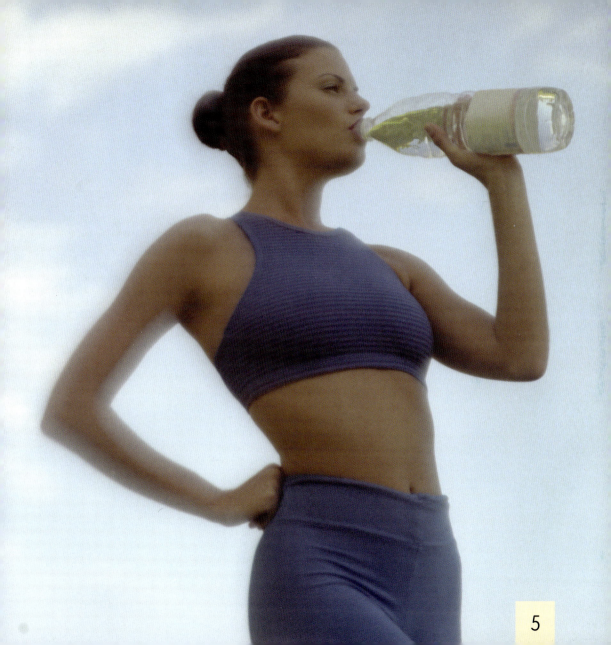

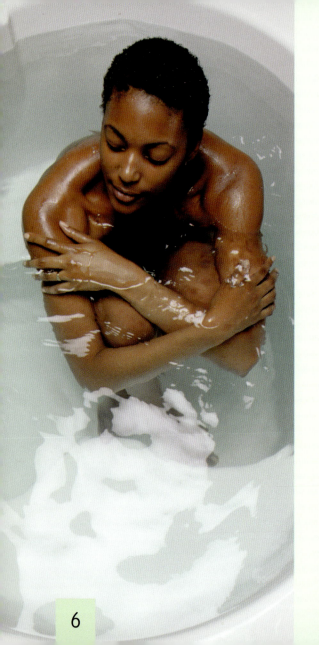

why
detox?

Throughout history, detox has been a way of life: from native Africans ritually consuming concoctions of sulphur and herbs in order to cleanse their systems of toxins and parasites, to Cleopatra bathing in milk to purify her skin, assisting with her famous youthful looks.

So why should we rid our bodies of toxins? If it is so important, why is it that those who don't, don't appear to suffer?

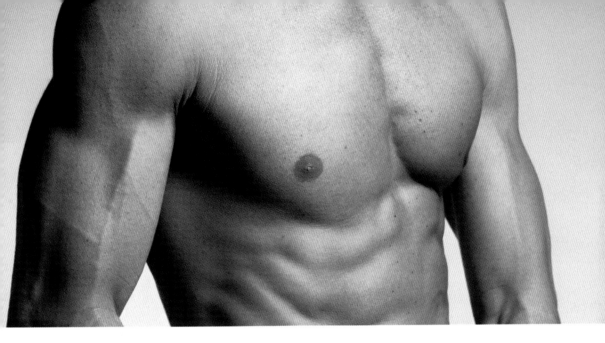

To answer the latter, it has been proven that our bodies can run on processed modified foods, but at what expense? Our body is like a finely-tuned engine; feed it with pure fuel and we get the optimum performance, feed it with the cheaper, less beneficial alternative, and it will under-perform. So it is clear why we should make a habit of detoxing. We shouldn't be satisfied with tiredness and depression being just "one of those things". The world is an exciting one, and something as simple as providing our body with the right fuel could help us achieve the things that we have always wanted to do.

Medical research has shown a correlation between the rise in asthma and cancer with the rise in pollution. The findings are out there, so what can we do? Airborne pollutants are inescapable so what viable option do we have? These toxins can be expelled from our bodies provided that our bodies are nutritionally fuelled to the optimum.

Centuries ago, the life expectancy was around forty. This was due to many reasons. Medical research wasn't what it is today, neither was plumbing, and sewage control problems caused a whole host of diseases. However, interestingly, people "existed" on the minimum nutritionally.

With a better immune system, and a more beneficial diet, could those people have survived into their sixties or even seventies? Looking to nature and the animal kingdom, the supply of fresh, unpolluted water and plants may contribute to the long life spans of certain animals, for example the African elephant. With the highest life expectancy in the animal kingdom perhaps we can deduce a link between the elephant's life span and diet?

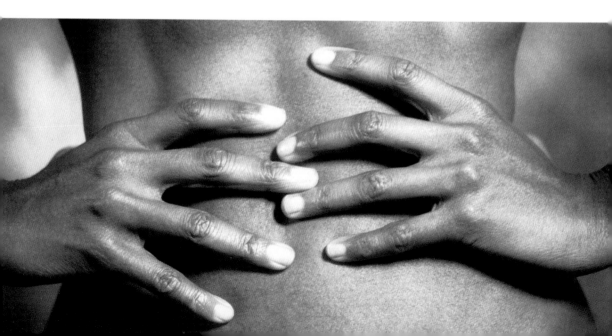

A well-fueled body not only creates the optimum physical benefits, but also provides us with a healthier state of mind. Who hasn't heard that old saying "Healthy body, healthy mind"? But who among us actually believes it? Chemicals that we ingest have been linked with the promotion of depression. An excess of aluminum, for example, has been suggested as a factor in the cause of Alzheimer's. So perhaps it is time to reassess our diet and realize the implications of what we ingest.

So finally, why should we detox? It is simply because the benefits of detox, although often small, are nonetheless significant. Physically, we can walk that extra mile, we can come home from work and get on with those niggling jobs that we all put off. Detox can also help combat depression and help us become more focussed. Perhaps most importantly, a revitalized immune system will allow us to lead a healthier life.

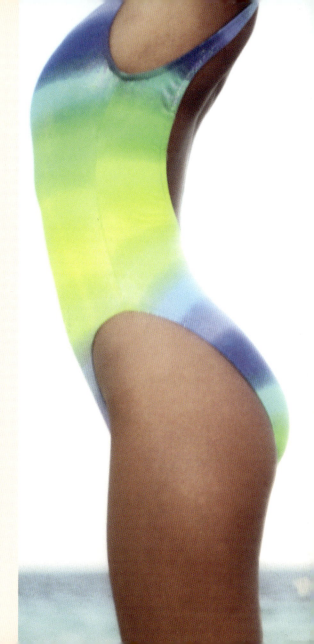

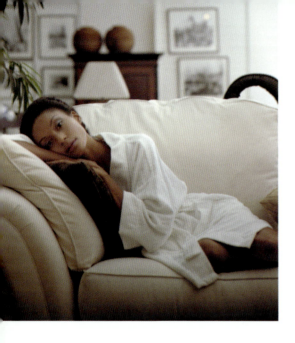

are you
in need of a detox?

Answer the following questions. The more you answer with a "yes", the more you will need a detox.

As a general rule:
If you answer "yes" to less than four questions then you probably don't need to detox. Between five and ten, then your body would benefit greatly from a detox. Should you say "yes" to more than ten, then you could be putting your body under enormous stress and this detox plan is strongly recommended.

- do you have dark circles under your eyes?
- do you suffer from headaches or migraines?
- is your skin spotty or dull?
- do you suffer from skin rashes or eczema?
- is your hair dull?
- do you suffer from joint or muscle aches and pains?
- do you suffer from sinus problems, catarrh or a stuffy nose?
- do you often have a bitter taste in your mouth?
- do you sweat a lot?
- do you suffer from stress?
- do you suffer from irritable bowel syndrome?
- do you suffer from flatulence?

- do you suffer from bloating?
- are you constantly tired?
- do you have difficulty maintaining concentration?
- do you have problems sleeping?
- do you suffer from mood swings, anxiety or depression?
- do you have cellulite?
- do you sometimes suffer from ear infections, earache or ringing in the ears?

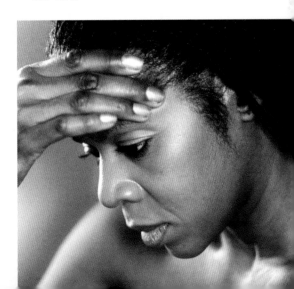

body works

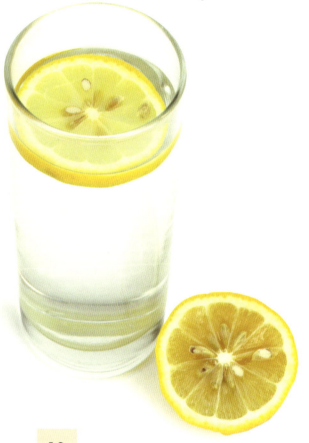

Being bombarded with toxins and other unwanted substances on a daily basis, can lead to both long- and short-term illness, as well as general ill health.

Our bodies are designed to deal with these problems, but if we do not take care, then things can start to go wrong, and our natural defense mechanisms soon start to fail.

the digestive system

The human body is a fascinating subject, the digestive system being one of its most amazing elements. As we all know, although we eat to survive most of us treat certain foods as a luxury. These luxuries, however, are usually the most problematic for us to digest!

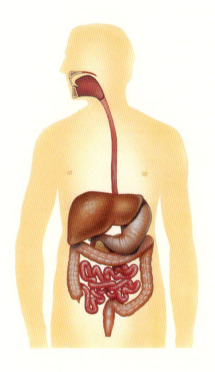

The digestive system processes the food we eat, to provide us with the vital nutrients that help our bodies to run smoothly. The stomach and intestine are the primary organs for absorbing these nutrients into the body. The secretion of acids and chemicals in these organs is vital to this process. We just have to do the easy part and eat the right foods in order for these chemicals and acids to be produced.

Food is broken down by digestive enzymes and "friendly" bacteria in the gut. If we have a poor diet, are stressed, taking antibiotics or have an excess of toxins, then our digestive systems will not function properly. Food can remain only partially digested and problems such as irritable bowel syndrome, constipation, nausea and bloating arise. This toxic undigested food can then leak into the bloodstream and cause other problems.

To keep the digestive system healthy, do not drink too much with a meal as this can dilute the digestive fluids. Only eat when hungry and try not to over-eat. Chew food slowly, and properly. Start the day with a glass of hot water and lemon juice, as this will boost your digestive system and prepare you for the day ahead.

the liver

Almost everything that enters the body passes through the liver. One of its functions is to remove toxins from the bloodstream. Harmful substances are neutralized here and passed on to the intestines in bile. The liver is also responsible for supplying energy to the body, by converting the energy from food into nutrients used by our cells. One of the problems we have if the liver is not functioning effectively is that it stores toxins, and also deposits them in fat cells. This can cause quite serious problems such as diabetes and cirrhosis.

To maintain a healthy liver, we should eat plenty of fresh fruit and vegetables, avoid processed, fried, sugary or salty foods, and cut down on alcohol and caffeine. If you do suffer from a sluggish liver, try supplementing your diet with the antioxidants vitamin C and E, selenium and betacarotene.

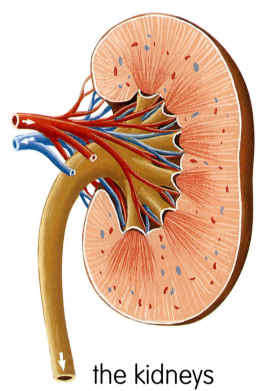

the kidneys

The kidneys filter toxins in the blood and eliminate them in urine. They also regulate the amount of fluid in the body and recycle nutrients. They need plenty of fresh water to function properly.

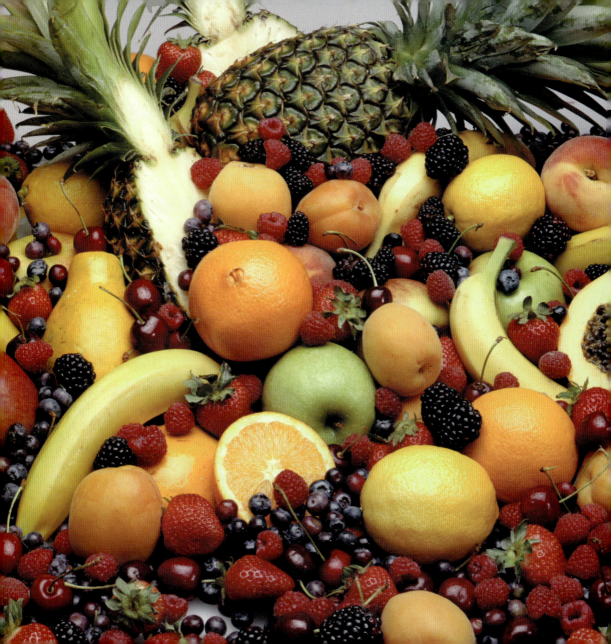

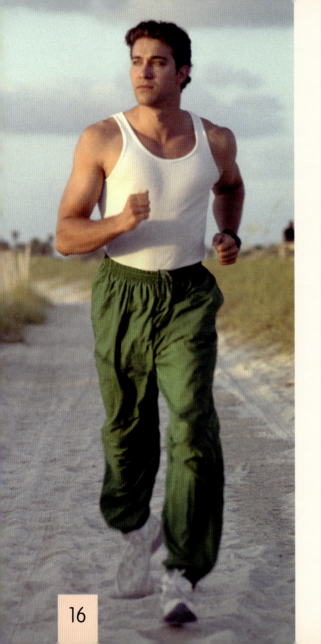

the skin

The body's largest organ, the skin, eliminates waste through the pores. Sweat and the sebaceous glands help to remove toxins. When we are unhealthy, this normally shows as a dull, lifeless complexion, with spots, blemishes, or rashes.

To keep your skin healthy, get plenty of sleep, fresh air, and exercise. Regular skin brushing will also help. Eat plenty of raw fruit and vegetables.

the lymphatic system

This system carries waste, toxins, dead cells and excess fluid to the lymph nodes, where the waste is filtered before being passed into the bloodstream. It is believed that if there are high levels of toxins present in the body then the lymphatic system will be slowed down.

This is shown in the form of cellulite, poor circulation and a weakened immune system. Massage helps to encourage a healthy lymphatic system, as does skin brushing, and exercise.

the lungs

Our lungs deal with airborne pollutants. Oxygen enters our bloodstream via the lungs, and waste, such as carbon dioxide, is removed via them. If we suffer from catarrh, blocked sinuses, or a constant runny nose, these are often signs of a problem with the respiratory system; we may not be inhaling enough oxygen or expelling all the waste gases.

We need to breathe correctly by slowly inhaling through the nose, filling our lungs. If we are breathing correctly, the lower part of the stomach should rise first, followed by the chest, and the breath should be slowly exhaled through the nostrils.

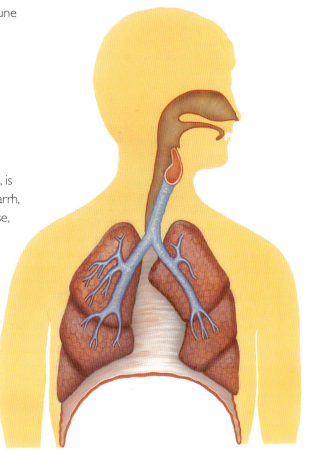

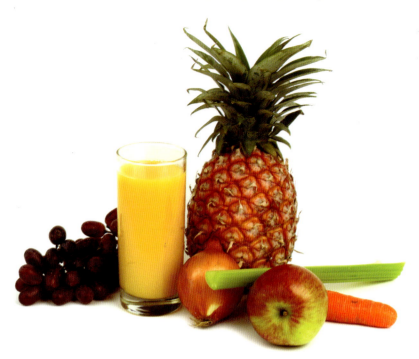

safety tips

Detoxing can create changes in the body. It is generally not advisable for people with ill health to embark on a long process of detoxification, unless done gradually, for example, by slowly cutting down on beverages that have high levels of caffeine, such as tea, coffee, or cola, eating more fresh fruit and vegetables, and drinking plenty of fresh fruit juices and water.

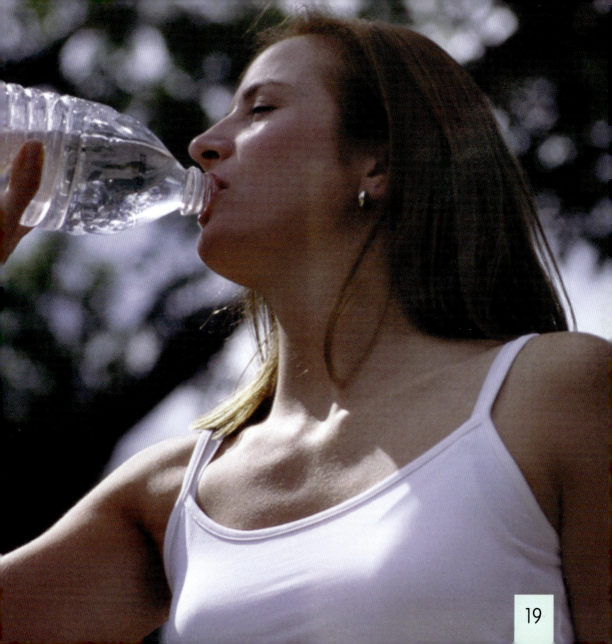

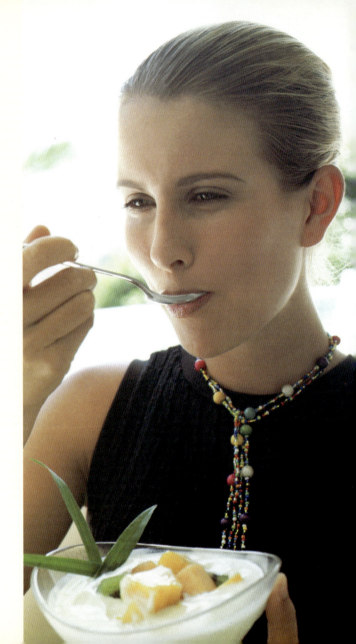

If you are in doubt about any aspect of healthy eating, detoxing or exercise, then your doctor is there to help. Never start something that you are unsure about without checking first. Your health is the most important thing you've got, so look after it and reap the rewards.

It is not recommended to detox without first consulting your doctor if you are:

- diabetic
- on prescribed medication
- being treated for a serious illness, such as cancer, liver disease, heart disease, or blood disorder
- pregnant

Although a doctor may normally recommend a healthy eating plan, remember detoxification can be intense and extreme caution is often advised.

Generally, making small, positive changes to your diet is beneficial to your health. Try to include parts of the detox plan in your day-to-day routine, such as drinking hot water and lemon juice in the morning, and drinking at least eight glasses of water per day. If the body doesn't have to struggle to remove harmful toxins, then it can function more efficiently, hopefully resulting in less illness and disease.

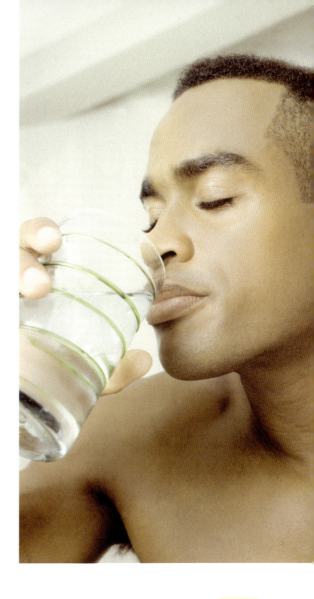

coping with
side effects

Detoxing can have powerful effects on the body as all the toxic waste is flushed out of your organs and fat tissue. This can cause some unpleasant side effects that you should be ready to deal with. These can include:

headaches

These usually affect coffee drinkers, as they can suffer from caffeine withdrawal. The effects usually only last 2-3 days. Usually, when the effects have worn off, the outcome is a much clearer head, which normally lasts until you start to drink beverages high in caffeine again. This suggests that, in the long term, caffeine has a detrimental effect on your health. Plenty of natural fruit juices, herbal teas, and water will help to keep headaches to a minimum. Another good remedy is one drop of lavender oil, dabbed on the temples.

skin eruptions

As the skin is a good detoxifier and a lot of waste is flushed out here, you can expect to come up in unsightly spots, blemishes and rashes. This normally lasts for about a week, but when they have cleared, the skin will be glowing and radiant. Using one of the natural face-mask recipes found in this book should help combat any nasty eruptions.

bad breath

Again this isn't very pleasant, but it is a sign that toxins are leaving your body. One theory is that it occurs when the body starts using its stores of fat, as this is where a lot of toxins are stored. A good remedy is peppermint tea which, as well as being refreshing and stimulating to the digestive system, helps to freshen the breath.

weight loss

Not an unpleasant side effect! During a two-day detox you can expect to lose up to 4 lb (1.8 kg). This is largely water, but a longer detox will affect fat stores. This is not a bad side effect, as any water loss is replaced with a good intake of fluids.

If you are serious about losing weight then a detox is the perfect way to start a sensible eating and exercise regime.

It is important to remember that these side effects are only temporary, following a good detox plan. Your body will soon combat them, and the end result will be a healthier and fitter person!

Warning:
Should any of these symptoms persist, consult your doctor.

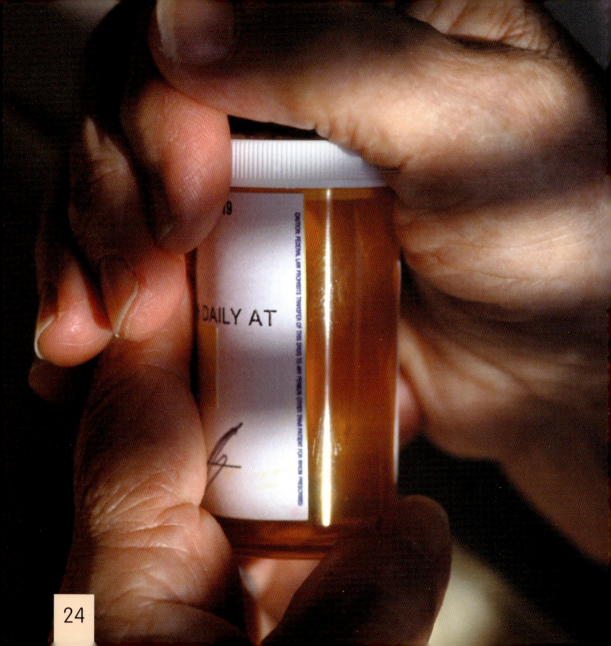

detox and
diets

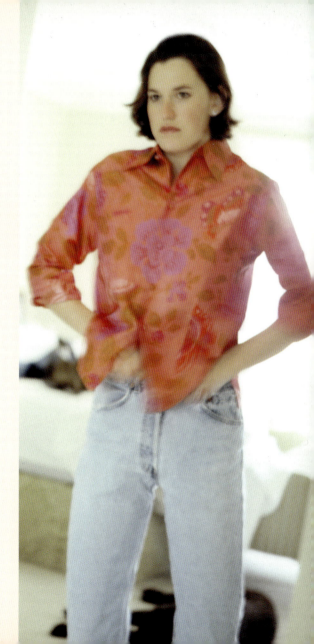

There are hundreds of diets, from cabbage diets, to egg diets, and low fat diets. If you need to lose weight, nutritionally-balanced meals and exercise may not produce overnight success but in the long term you will be a healthy weight. That is the only dieting advice you will receive in this book.

Detoxing is a regime to combat all the harmful toxins in your body, not an attempt to lose fat cells. Hopefully, by now you will be aware of how your body is affected by toxins. So when you have a headache, don't take that asprin! When you are lethargic and mentally tired, don't lie down in front of the TV. Your body is giving you the warning signals, so don't ignore them or take medication to cover up the symptoms, just detox!

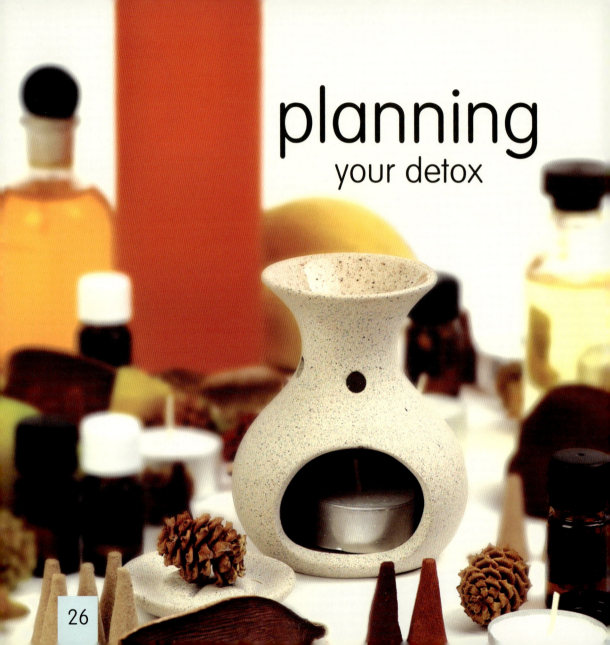

Before beginning your detox, be warned that for however long you practice this plan you will encounter various changes. These are the various side effects outlined on page 22, so try to prepare for all eventualities.

The body has often been likened to the structure of a house. Clear out the attic of your house and the supporting walls will not be put under so much pressure, i.e. clear your mind of all your worries and problems, "lift the weight off your shoulders," and concentrate on what is to take place.

Spring cleaning your home is one place to start your detox. You should try to think of this plan as an opportunity to cleanse both yourself, and your surroundings. Before you begin your detox, make a mental note of your state of mind and your state of health. When you have completed your plan, compare your notes and see the improvements. When you are mentally prepared, take action by throwing out all foods that will hinder your progress. Without willpower, you will not succeed. Don't be fooled into thinking that even a one-day detox will be easy. On a typical day how many meals do you have, how many snacks? You may be surprised at how much you actually eat.

Finally, create a haven inside your home. Fill a room with cushions, candles, and aromatherapy oils. Set up a stereo to play revitalizing music and just retreat and unwind. Make this a room where you can praise yourself for the hard work you have done and concentrate on how well you are treating your body.

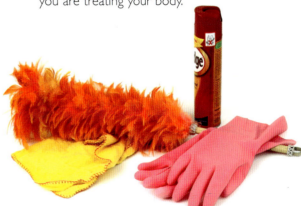

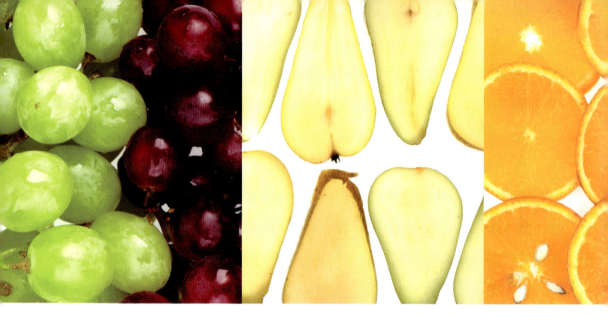

food and nutrition

Once you have decided on the length of your detox plan, you should write up a shopping list of all the things you will need.

It may sound easier than you think, but remember, you have to walk past the aisles with the chips, chocolate, and candy bars and all the other junky snack foods that you should be avoiding!

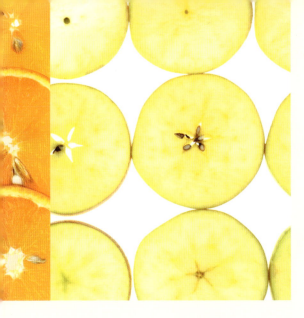

fruit

Fruit is a powerful detox food. It supplies the body with numerous vitamins, minerals and antioxidants, along with fiber and a good supply of energy. Fruit is an excellent cleanser; fruit pectin has been shown to bind with heavy metals and fruit fiber with toxins, flushing them out of the body. Organic produce is best, but if this is not available, make sure you wash all fruit before eating to remove any residues of pesticides.

apples

These have a high fiber and pectin content, along with vitamin C, betacarotene, and fructose for energy. Their fruit acids also aid digestion, and help to remove toxins from the liver.

pears

A high water content makes pears a good diuretic. They also contain vitamin C, potassium, fiber and pectin.

grapes

These have a very high antioxidant content and are powerful detoxifiers.

oranges

High in the antioxidant vitamin C, oranges help to protect against free radicals. They also stimulate the digestive system, and help reduce the risk of heart disease and cancer.

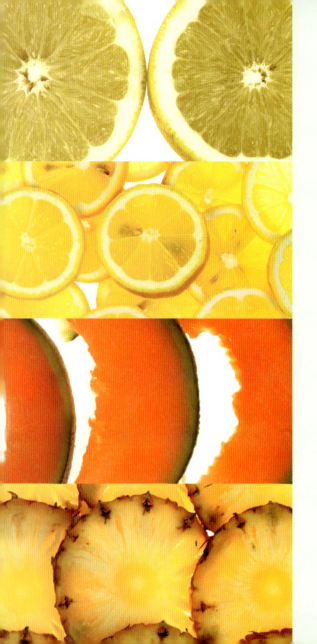

grapefruits

These are packed full of vitamin C, betacarotene, calcium, potassium, and phosphorus. Eat at the start of a meal to help stimulate digestion.

lemons

You should start off any day with a glass of hot water with freshly squeezed lemon juice. The juice is a powerful cleanser and antiseptic and stimulates the liver and gall bladder.

melons

The melon is another fruit that has a very high water content, making it excellent for the kidneys and digestive system. It is high in vitamin C and betacarotene.

pineapples

The fresh fruit contains the antibacterial enzyme bromelain, which is destroyed in

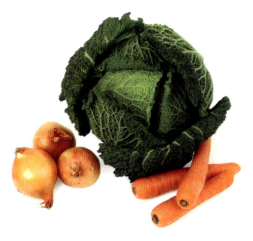

the canning process. These are very rich in vitamin C, folic acid, and also contain calcium, magnesium and potassium.

vegetables

Just as fruits have a powerful effect on the body, so too, do vegetables. Containing a vast array of nutrients, they are also packed with bioflavonoids, and other phytochemicals which help the body's systems. Most of the following vegetables are best eaten raw or juiced to retain their natural nutrients. Again, organic is best, but if this is not available, ensure that you wash the vegetable properly before eating.

onions

Onions contain antiviral and antibacterial nutrients which protect the body. They are a good source of the antioxidant quercetin, which has been shown to lower blood pressure, and help in fighting cancer. Garlic, which is part of the same family, has a powerful boost on the immune system.

carrots

These are one of the best detoxifying vegetables and contain large amounts of betacarotene, which has been found to lower the risk of cancer.

cabbages

Rich in betacarotene, vitamins C and E, folate, thiamine, potassium, and iron, the cabbage is also rich in antiviral and antibacterial nutrients. It aids digestion, cleanses the liver and detoxifies the stomach and upper bowels.

celery

This is an important detox food as it is a good diuretic and laxative.

tomatoes

Contain high levels of vitamins C and E, betacarotene, calcium, phosphorus and magnesium. They are reputed to aid the liver and help reduce inflammation caused by cirrhosis.

broccoli

This is high on the list of vegetables that have a powerful detoxing effect. Broccoli contains cancer-fighting phytochemicals and also supplies vitamins C and B, calcium, zinc, folate, iron, and potassium.

beetroot

Reputed to be one of the best liver cleansers, beetroot is another powerful

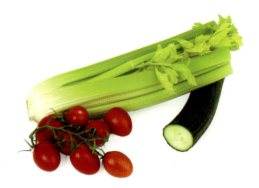

detoxifier. It contains high levels of vitamin C and betacarotene, and also calcium and iron.

cucumber

With a high water content, this is a very effective diuretic, thus assisting the kidneys to eliminate waste.

oils

A certain amount of fat is essential to our diet. The problem is most people eat the wrong types. Unrefined, cold-pressed oils such as sunflower, rapeseed, and extra-virgin olive oil contain essential fatty acids and vitamin E.

beans and pulses

These provide good amounts of protein, fiber, vitamins, and minerals and are low in fat. Beans also contain phytoestrogens, which are reputed to protect against certain cancers.

grains

Wholegrains and cereals are low in fat, contain a good source of protein, carbohydrates, fiber, vitamins, and minerals. Grains to include in your detox plan are brown rice, barley, couscous, oats, corn, and quinoa. Wheat should be avoided as it is a common allergen. Unprocessed wholegrains should be used as they retain most of their nutrients.

nuts and seeds

A small amount of nuts should be eaten daily as these are packed with vitamin E, B vitamins, iron, magnesium, calcium, phosphorus, potassium, and essential fatty acids. The downside is the high fat content, so they should be eaten in moderation. The most nutritious are almonds, cashews, chestnuts, hazelnuts, and walnuts.

Seeds such as sunflower, sesame, pumpkin, and linseed are rich in vitamin E and omega 6 fatty acids. These help to support the immune system.

Sprouted beans, seeds, and grains contain an even greater amount of vitamins and minerals. These can be bought in grocery stores, health food stores, or grown at home.

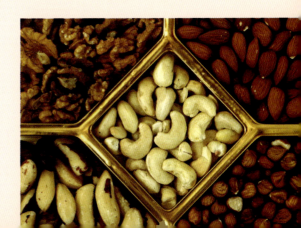

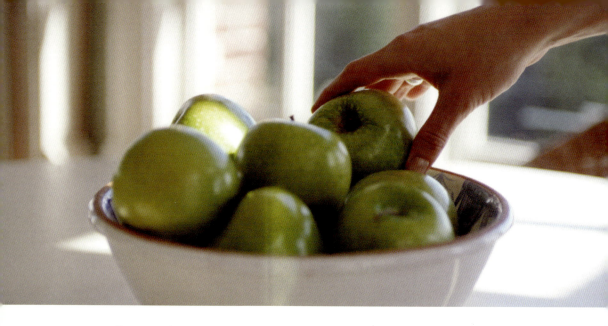

foods to eat

Eating five or more portions of fruit and vegetables a day can reduce the risk of diseases such as heart disease and some cancers. This is due to fruit and vegetables containing almost all the essential vitamins and minerals needed to boost all the body's systems. A plate of cabbage, cauliflower, and broccoli would be very nutritious followed by a fresh carrot and tomato juice. However, healthy as it may be, it hasn't got the appeal of a chocolate gâteau! But, fruit and vegetables do not have to be boring and the recipes in this book (page 58) will show that healthy food can be fun too.

Make sure you drink plenty of water, to help flush out the toxins that make the liver work overtime.

Remember the largest organ of the body is the skin. The more water we drink the more we sweat, and expel toxins. Six to eight glasses a day are recommended. Herbal teas are a good alternative as they have the added bonus of calming your nerves, relaxing you, or settling your stomach.

During your detox, your immune system should be taken care of, for both your physical and mental well-being. Vitamin C is a good boost for your body. It helps produce white blood cells, which help to prevent viruses and disease. A healthy immune system can also help to prevent depression.

Organic food should be eaten wherever possible. Although more expensive, organic produce is generally considered to be far healthier and tastier than conventionally grown food. "Going organic" also takes away an unnecessary ingestion of chemicals.

The motto for choosing which food to eat is "If you feel you shouldn't, then don't!"

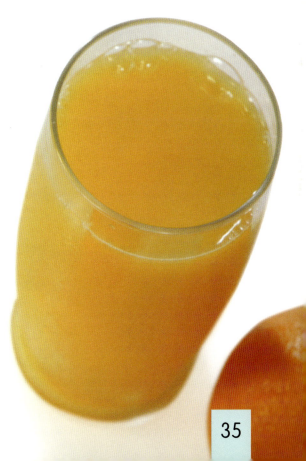

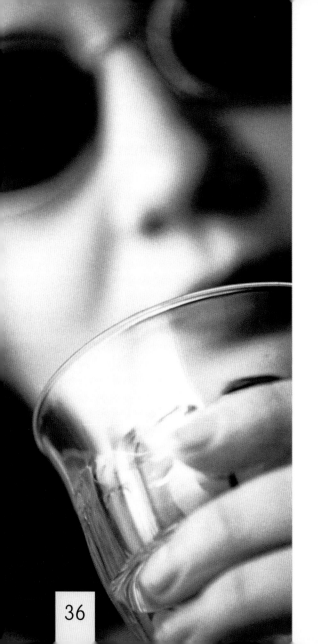

foods to avoid

Too much of a good thing is bad for you! Alcohol, if consumed in large quantities, can harm your liver.

The depletion of essential nutrients causes a higher risk of dehydration or, in the worst-case scenario, cirrhosis of the liver. Caffeine, another stimulant often taken to prevent tiredness, causes headaches, high blood pressure and, ironically, after a while will cause tiredness. Decaffeinated coffee and teas

Arguably, many chemicals are slowly sending us to an early grave. It is fair to say that we cannot escape them, but taken in small quantities, providing our vital organs are being nurtured, our bodies can cope.

are not as healthy as they seem, since the decaffeinating process takes place through chemicals being added to the drinks.

Margarine is seen as a healthier alternative to butter due to the reduction in saturated fat. However, during margarine production, chemicals are added to reduce the fat content. The saturated fats in butter and other dairy products slow down the lymphatic system, and can lead to clogged arteries.

Salt can cause high blood pressure and water retention in the kidneys. Sugar can cause a problem with blood sugar levels.

Flour-based products can cause many problems including wheat allergies, and the refining process also uses a lot of chemicals.

Non-organic meats or fish often contain growth-promoting chemicals. Red meats are also connected with bowel cancer, due to the difficulties we have digesting them. Processed foods contain all types of chemicals that can destroy the nutritional benefits of natural ingredients.

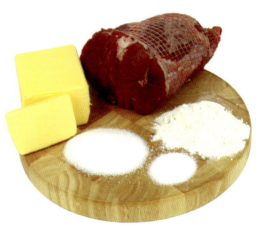

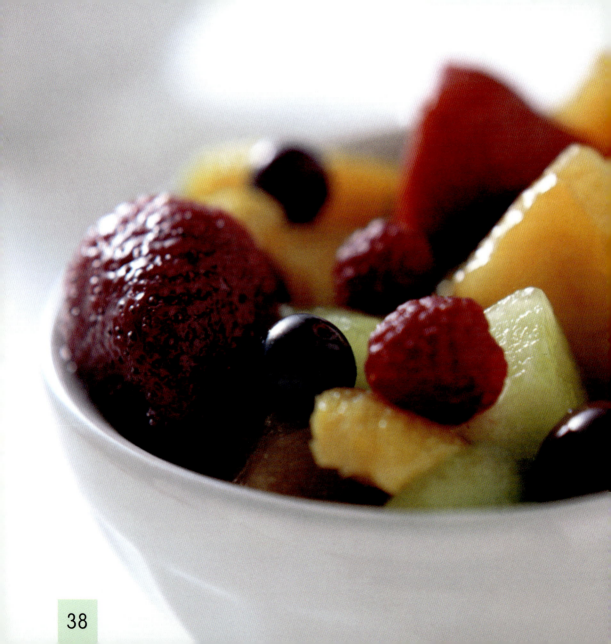

natural
supplements

As well as a diet filled with fresh fruit, vegetables and wholesome nutritious food, we can also assist our bodies with natural supplements.

aloe vera

This has immunity-boosting, antiviral and antibacterial properties. It is soothing on the digestive system and a good tonic.

antioxidants

These are found in most fresh fruit and vegetables. They detoxify harmful "free radicals", which can trigger cancers, inflammation, arterial damage, and aging. Antioxidants include essential vitamins and minerals such as vitamins A, C, and E, betacarotene, zinc, selenium, and many other non-essential supplements such as milk thistle, blueberry extract, bioflavonoids, and lipoic acid.

cat's claw

From the Peruvian rainforest plant, this is a powerful antiviral antioxidant and also boosts the immune system.

garlic

For those that do not like the taste or smell of garlic, odorless garlic tablets are available. The benefits of garlic are great; not only does it have antiviral, antibacterial and antifungal properties, it is also rich in amino acids and antioxidants.

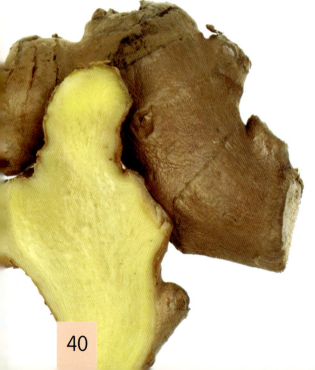

ginger

You may notice ginger in some of the juice recipes, this is due to its soothing effect on the digestive system. It is also good for the circulatory system.

probiotics

These are beneficial, or "friendly" bacteria that live in the digestive system. They help to maintain balance and can fight off stomach infections. These can be taken in tablet form, although they exist in natural yoghurt. They are highly beneficial when a course of antibiotics, which destroy "friendly" bacteria, has been taken.

selenium

Selenium is an important antioxidant, but is becoming less available in our foods, as we rely on artificial fertilizers and chemicals, which destroy this nutrient.

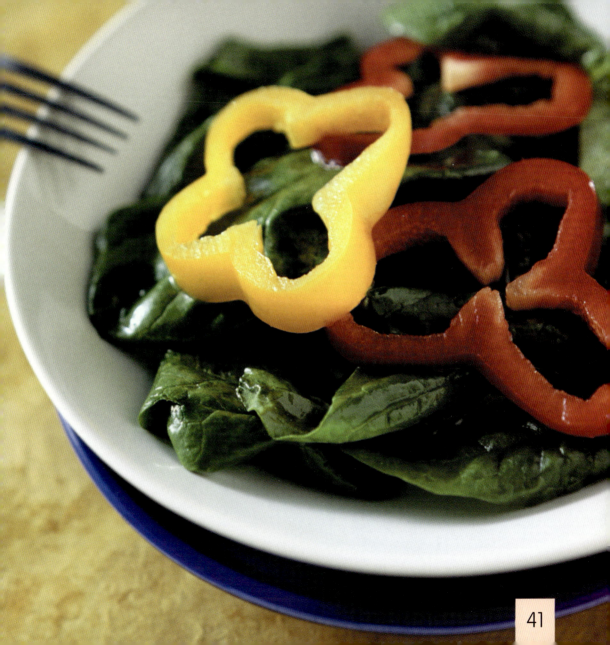

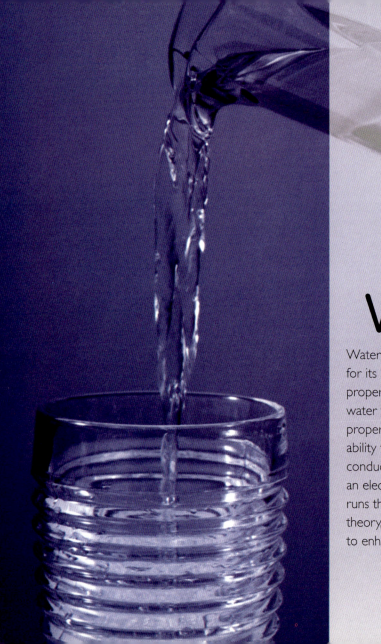

water

Water has always been recognized for its soothing, calming, and cleansing properties. There are many uses of water that have various effects. One property that all water has is the ability to be magnetized and to conduct electricity. Our bodies have an electromagnetic energy field that runs through and around them. In theory, water can harness this energy to enhance relaxation and healing.

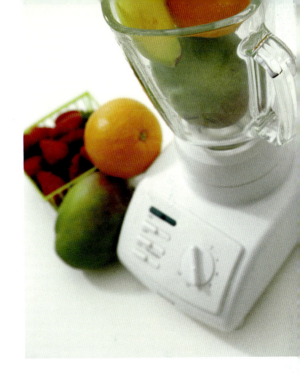

The human body is made up of approximately 75 percent water, present in all of our tissues, and therefore we need to ensure that we drink at least eight glasses of water per day. Not only does this stop us from becoming dehydrated, but it also ensures that toxins are flushed out of our systems, it helps to regulate body temperature, it supplies the body with oxygen and nutrients, and it aids muscle cells in producing energy.

As water from the faucet can contain additional chemicals, mineral or filtered water is better. However, beware of bottled spring water, as this may just be another form of faucet water! Distilled water should be avoided as this leeches all the essential minerals from the body!

Do not be misled into thinking that you are getting the correct amount of fluids by drinking eight cups of tea or coffee per day. These have a diuretic effect on the body, causing in dehydration. So too do drinks high in refined sugar. Natural fruit juices can count as part of your intake.

The need to drink at least eight glasses per day cannot be stressed enough. You will not only feel more energetic, but you will see the difference, with glowing skin and glossy hair.

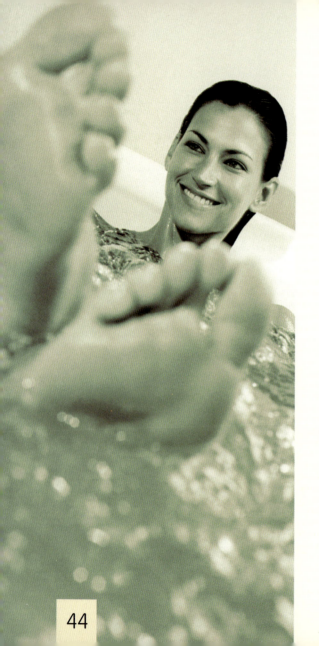

water
treatments

mineral water

In early Victorian Britain, the use of mineral water became very popular, and many mineral baths were established. The Romans, too, were well aware of the relaxing nature of these baths and often built cities around such places (for example, Bath in England). Throughout the world, natural mineral springs flow, making a very concentrated mixture of the Earth's vital elements available.

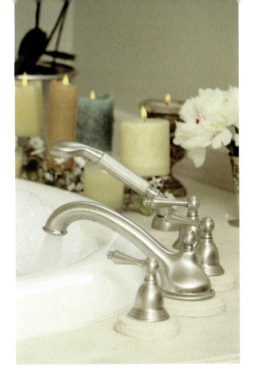

salt water

The ocean stands apart from other waters because of its salt content. The Dead Sea is so heavy with salt that you can only float in it! Many people who have muscular or rheumatic symptoms bathe in salt water as it draws out impurities and reduces pain. All salt water has the effect of cleansing through the skin, partially due to the natural process of osmosis. "Osmotic pressure" is the tendency of any fluid to draw from the "least dense" to the "most dense". Since salt water is too dense to enter the membrane, it attempts to balance itself by drawing towards it the lighter fluid properties from within the body. It can act as an excellent anti-inflammatory, as well as relieving tired muscles and joints.

One of the best ways we can experience this at home is by having an Epsom salts bath. The salts are magnesium sulfate, which creates a static electrified field in

Bathing in these waters should be done with great care as their penetrating qualities can affect the internal balance of the body. Their detoxifying properties are excellent as they promote the opening of the skin's pores, thereby allowing toxins to be flushed out.

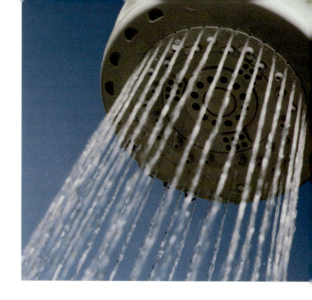

the water. When we are immersed in this water it creates a magnetic balance. Magnesium sulfate also draws out excess sodium, phosphorus and nitrogenous toxins from the body.

Pour 1 lb of Epsom salts into a warm bath and soak for twenty minutes. Afterward pat yourself dry and go to bed or relax for an hour. You may sweat during the night, so make sure you drink plenty of water before you retire. In the morning, have a bath or shower to remove any salt residues. This form of hydrotherapy helps speed up the detoxification process.

other water treatments

Another water treatment that you can do at home is a Sitz bath. Spend a few minutes in a warm bath and then have a very brief cold shower or bath. The change in temperature will stimulate the circulation and encourage the removal of toxins.

This can also be done in the shower. Take a warm shower until your skin is warm and glowing. Then turn off the hot water and direct the cold water onto your face and down your body. This should last about thirty seconds, and then get out of the shower, dry yourself off and keep warm. Again, this helps stimulate the circulation.

sauna and steam bath

These encourage perspiration and boost circulation, which aids the removal of toxins. Spend only 5-10 minutes at a time in the sauna, and take a cold shower in between. Always finish with a cold shower.

Most of us don't have the luxury of a home sauna, but the following can give us a similar effect.

Run a bath to about 105-110°F (40-43°C), this is just above body temperature. Use a thermometer to check the temperature. Lie in the bath for 15-20 minutes with your whole body immersed and just your head sticking out of the water. When you have finished, wrap yourself in a warm towel to dry off and go and lie down and relax for another twenty minutes.

aromatherapy

Run a warm bath and add a few drops of your favorite essential oils, or a ready-mixed blend of aromatherapy oil. Choose oils you immediately like the smell of to help you relax further. Calming oils include camomile, lavender, sandalwood, and patchouli. Stimulating oils include rosemary, geranium, and rose. Juniper has a particularly detoxifying effect.

Warning
If you suffer from any type of heart disease, avoid these baths. If you suffer from eczema or high blood pressure, avoid the Epsom bath.

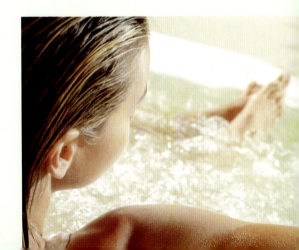

herbal teas

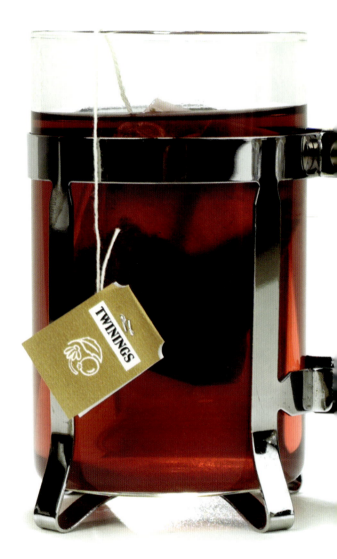

People have used herbal teas for centuries, for medicinal use, and for enjoyment as tasty and refreshing beverages. Not all herbs are suitable for making tea, so be informed on each particular herb before drinking a tea made from it.

Herbal teas are ideal during a detox, as well as for daily drinking, as they are caffeine-free, count towards your daily fluid intake and, most importantly, are packed full of health-giving herbs.

The following are a selection of some of the best pre-blended herbal teas from Twinings, and some of the more popular herbs you can use at home. Similar blends will be available from other companies.

echinacea and raspberry

Echinacea is a very powerful antibacterial and antiviral herb, which was commonly used by Native American Indians as an antidote to snake venom. Today it is used to treat all manner of infections, especially colds, flu, and sore throats. Raspberry is excellent for digestive problems, and has good healing properties.

peppermint

Peppermint is an excellent digestive herb, good for stomach pains, dyspepsia, colic, nausea, and easing symptoms of colds.

camomile, honey and vanilla

This is a very relaxing tea. Honey has good antibacterial properties and is calming on the digestive system. Vanilla is mainly used as a flavoring, but traditionally it is used in herbal medicine as an emollient balm.

camomile and spiced apple

Camomile and spiced apple is a great winter warmer. Camomile is renowned for its relaxing properties. It is also excellent for digestive problems as it is settling and soothing.

Apple is a good detoxifier and is full of antioxidants, antibacterial, and antiviral properties. The mixed spices in this tea make it ideal during times of colds and flu.

lemon and ginger

The lemon has an abundance of positive properties and is the most valuable of all fruits for preserving health. During colds and flu, it can keep fevers in check. It is a particularly good diuretic, which is ideal during a detox. It is also reputed to ease the symptoms of acute rheumatism.

Ginger is a favorite in both Western and Chinese herbal medicine for digestive problems. It is used to relieve colic, gastritis and dyspepsia. It is also good during colds and flu.

You can buy herbal tea bags in all sorts of varieties, or you could make your own herbal tea:

Add two tablespoons of fresh, or one tablespoon of dried herb (or crushed seed) to the pot for each cup of water, plus an extra two tablespoons of fresh, or one tablespoon of dried, "for the pot".

Pour boiling water over the herbs. Let them steep, covered, for about five minutes. This is not an exact timing, and you should check at varying intervals to find the right strength for your purposes, at which point you should strain the herbs out of the water and serve. Different herbs need different amounts of time to steep.

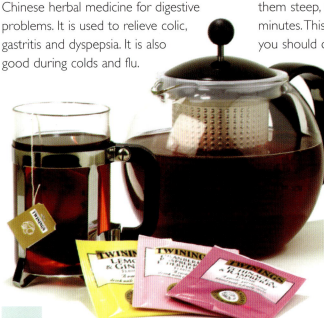

good herbs to use

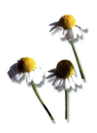

camomile
This is a good bedtime drink, as it has a soothing fragrance. It is also gentle on the urinary tract, and soothes any inflammation there.

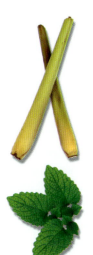

lemon grass
Good for the digestive system and also for helping to relieve headaches.

lemon balm
This can be quite a sedative drink, so it's best drunk at bedtime. It is also good during colds and flu, as it has excellent antiviral and antibacterial properties.

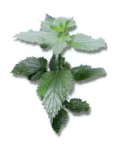

nettle
This has a very "herby" taste, so is not to everyone's taste, but it is recommended as a tonic. It is especially good if you are cutting out caffeine, as it helps to keep you alert.

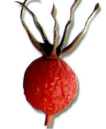

rose hip
Excellent during a cold as it helps to boost the immune system.

juices

Both fruit and vegetable juices are a vital part of detoxing. With a vast array of concentrated nutrients and antioxidants, freshly-squeezed juices encourage the elimination of toxins and stimulate the whole body, while being gentle on the digestive system. There are some great-tasting juices here, but you can always experiment with your own blends! The recipes make about two servings, and can be blended or juiced.

apple and melon
Good for removing toxins from the liver.

1 apple, peeled and cored
½ honeydew melon
4 oz (100 g) red grapes
4 tsp lemon juice

Cut the melon into quarters and remove the skin and seeds. Quarter the apple. Juice the fruit and add the lemon juice.

melon and pear
To stimulate the circulation.

½ galia melon
2 pears
1 in. (2.5 cm) piece of fresh ginger root

Quarter the melon and remove the seeds and skin. Quarter the pears. Juice all the ingredients.

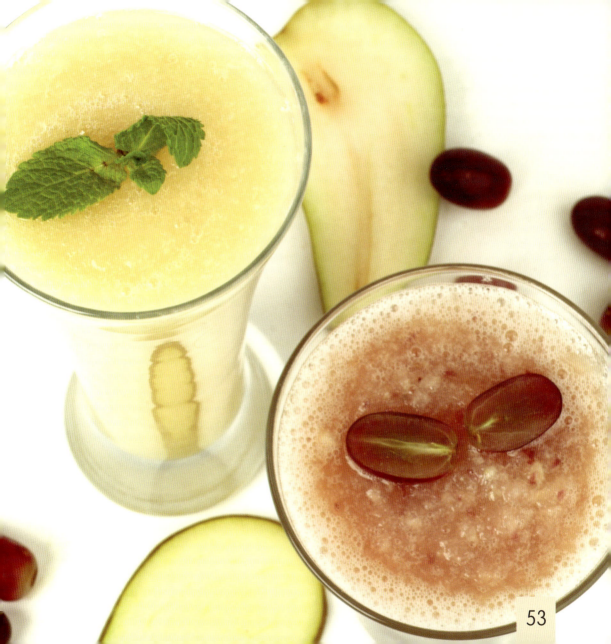

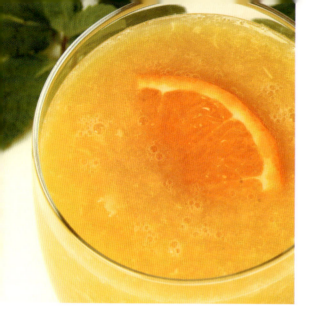

orange and grapefruit

Great boost for the immune system.

1 grapefruit
1 orange
2 tbsp lemon juice

Peel the grapefruit and orange and cut into segments. Juice the fruit and then stir in the lemon juice.

mango and pineapple

Good for the digestive system and kidneys.

1 small mango
½ pineapple

Peel the mango and cut away from the stone. Remove the pineapple skin and cut into chunks. Juice together.

tropical

Good for the liver and kidneys.

1 papaya
½ cantaloupe melon
4 oz (100 g) seedless white grapes

Skin and de-seed the papaya and cut into slices. Quarter the melon and remove the skin and seeds. Cut into chunks, add the grapes and juice all the ingredients.

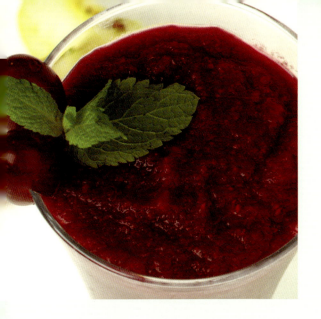
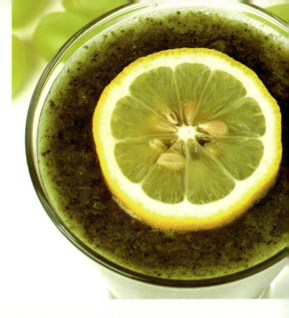

apple and carrot
A good liver cleanser and detoxifier.

2 apples, peeled and cored
1 large carrot
2 oz (50 g) cooked beetroot
4 oz (100 g) red grapes

Quarter the apples, top and tail the carrot. Juice the fruit and vegetables together.

apple and grape
Good for the kidneys, liver and skin.

1 apple, peeled and cored
5 oz (150 g) white grapes
1 oz (30 g) watercress
small handful of fresh coriander
1 tbsp lemon juice

Quarter the apple. Juice all the ingredients together.

red cabbage and apple

A natural diuretic, antiviral and antibacterial.

½ small red cabbage
2 apples, peeled and cored
½ fennel bulb
1 tbsp lemon juice

Quarter the apples. Slice the cabbage and fennel. Juice the fruit and vegetables together, then add the lemon juice.

apple carrot and orange

Good for arthritus sufferers.

3 carrots
1 apple, peeled and cored
1 orange

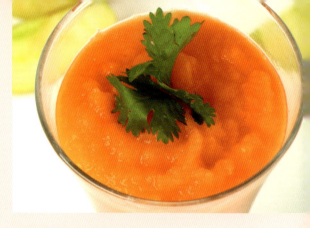

Quarter the apples. Top and tail the carrots. Peel the orange and cut into segments, and then juice all the ingredients together.

carrot and spinach

Good supply of antioxidants to help detox the system.

3 carrots
1 oz (25 g) spinach
4 oz (100 g) cooked beetroot
2 celery sticks

Top and tail the carrots, and juice all the vegetables together.

tomato and lettuce

Good for digestion, and full of nutrients.

3 large tomatoes
½ lettuce
¼ of a cucumber
handful of fresh parsley
1 tbsp lemon juice

Halve and quarter the tomatoes and lettuce. Peel and chop the cucumber. Juice all the ingredients.

strawberry and peach

Good for the skin.

2 cups of strawberries
1 peach

Hull the strawberries. Quarter the peach and pull out the stone. Juice the fruits.

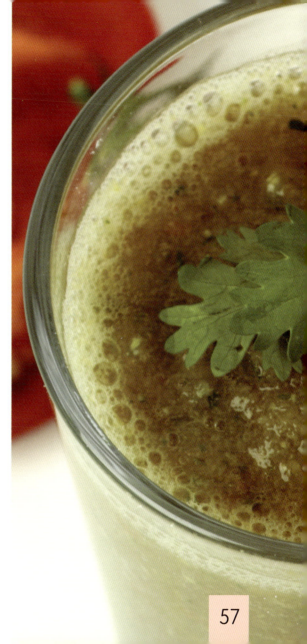

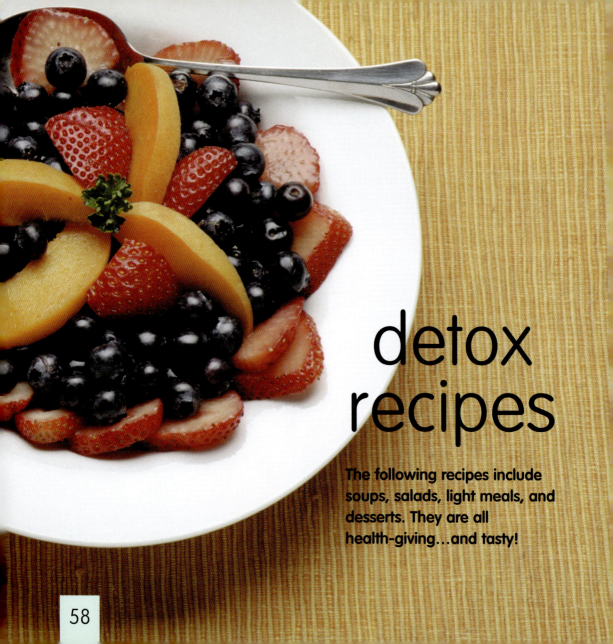

detox recipes

The following recipes include soups, salads, light meals, and desserts. They are all health-giving…and tasty!

soups

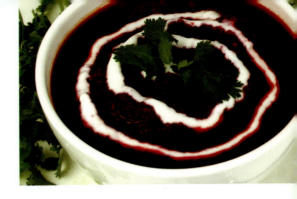

borsch

The main ingredient in this classic soup is beetroot, which is a very effective detoxifier, and cleanses the liver and kidneys. It is rich in antioxidants and iron.

Serves 4

2 lb (900 g) beetroot, peeled
2 carrots, peeled
2 celery sticks
2 onions, sliced
4 tomatoes, peeled, de-seeded and chopped
1 large parsley sprig
2 cloves
2 garlic cloves, crushed
4 whole peppercorns
2½ pints (1.2 liters) vegetable stock
freshly ground black pepper
3 tbsp olive oil

Cut the beetroot, carrots, and celery into fairly thick strips. Heat the oil in a large pan and cook the onions over a low heat for five minutes. Add the beetroot, carrots, and celery and cook for a further five minutes, stirring occasionally. Add the crushed garlic and chopped tomatoes to the pan and cook for two more minutes. Continue stirring.

Tie the parsley, cloves and peppercorns in a piece of muslin and add to the pan, along with the vegetable stock. Bring to the boil, cover and simmer for 1¼ hours, or until the vegetables are tender. Discard the bag of herbs, wait until cool enough, then blitz in the blender, stir in the pepper and gently reheat. Serve with a swirl of natural yoghurt if desired.

tomato and basil soup

This soup provides a large amount of antioxidants and aids digestion.

Serves 4

3 tbsp olive oil
1 finely chopped onion
2 lb (900 g) ripe plum tomatoes, chopped
1 garlic clove, chopped
3 pints (1½ liters) vegetable stock
2 tbsp tomato purée
2 tbsp shredded fresh basil
freshly ground pepper

Heat the oil in a large saucepan and add the onions. Cook gently for five minutes, stirring occasionally until softened but not brown. Stir in the tomatoes and garlic, and then add the stock, tomato purée and pepper. Bring to the boil, then lower the heat, half cover the pan and simmer gently for twenty minutes, stirring occasionally.

Transfer the soup to a food processor and add the basil. Process the ingredients. Press the blended soup through a sieve into a clean saucepan. Gently warm through before serving.

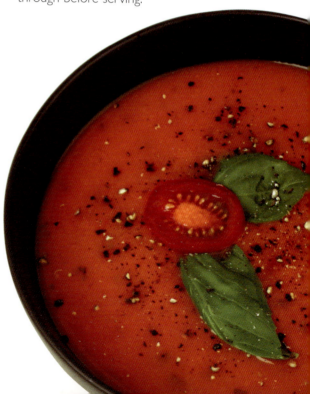

salads

bean salad with red pepper dressing

This is a good detox food and will provide a steady amount of energy.

Serves 4

1 large red pepper
1 large garlic clove, crushed
1 oz (25 g) fresh oregano leaves
1 tbsp lemon juice
4 tbsp olive oil
14 oz (400 g) canned flageolet beans, drained and rinsed
7 oz (200 g) canned cannellini beans, drained and rinsed
freshly ground black pepper

Preheat the oven to 200°C/400°F/gas mark 6. Place the red pepper on a baking sheet, brush with oil and roast for thirty minutes, or until soft. Remove the pepper from the oven and leave to cool. When the pepper is cool carefully peel off the skin. Rinse the peeled pepper under running water. Slice the pepper in half and remove the stem and seeds. Dice the pepper, retaining any juice, and set aside.

Heat the remaining olive oil in a saucepan and cook the garlic for about a minute until softened. Remove from the heat, then add the oregano and parsley, the roasted red pepper, and any retained juices and the lemon juice. Stir together.

Put the flageolet and cannellini beans in a large serving bowl and pour over the dressing. Season with the black pepper, and gently stir until combined. Serve warm.

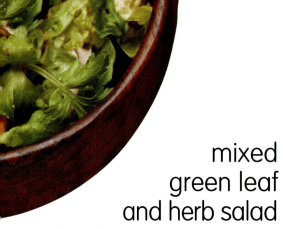

light meals

mixed green leaf and herb salad

Serves 4

½ oz (15 g) mixed fresh herbs such as dill, basil, parsley, mint, sorrel, fennel, coriander and chervil
12 oz (350 g) mixed salad leaves such as rocket, chicory, watercress, radicchio, curly endive, and oakleaf lettuce
1½ fl oz (50 ml) extra-virgin olive oil
1 tbsp cider vinegar
freshly ground black pepper

Wash and dry the herbs and salad leaves. In a bowl, blend the olive oil, cider vinegar, and pepper. Place the salad leaves and herbs in another bowl and mix well. Drizzle with the dressing to serve.

brown rice risotto with mushrooms

This is a good source of B vitamins and is rich in fiber.

Serves 4

9 oz (250 g) brown long grain rice
½ oz (15 g) dried porcini mushrooms
1 tbsp olive oil
4 shallots, finely chopped
2 garlic cloves, crushed
100 ml (3½ fl oz) vegetable stock
1 lb (450 g) mixed mushrooms, quartered
2 tbsp chopped fresh parsley
freshly ground black pepper

Place the dried porcini mushrooms in a bowl and cover with 5 fl oz (150 ml) hot water. Leave to soak for at least twenty minutes, until the mushrooms are rehydrated. Heat the oil in a large saucepan, add the shallots and garlic, and cook gently for five minutes, stirring occasionally.

Drain the porcini, retaining the liquid, and chop.

Add the brown rice to the shallot mixture and stir to coat the grains in the oil. Stir in the vegetable stock and the porcini liquid into the rice mixture in the saucepan. Bring to the boil, lower the heat and simmer, uncovered, for twenty minutes or until most of the liquid has been absorbed, stirring frequently.

Add all the mushrooms, mix well and cook the risotto for a further 10-15 minutes until the liquid has been absorbed. Season with freshly ground pepper and stir in the chopped parsley. Serve immediately.

mixed vegetable casserole

Serves 4

1 eggplant
8 oz (225 g) fresh or frozen peas
8 oz (225 g) green beans cut into
   1 in. (2.5 cm) pieces
4 zucchini cut into ½ in. (1 cm) strips
2 onions, finely chopped
1 lb (450 g) potatoes, diced
1 red pepper, seeded and sliced
14 oz (400 g) chopped canned tomatoes
5 fl oz (150 ml) vegetable stock
4 tbsp olive oil
1 tsp paprika

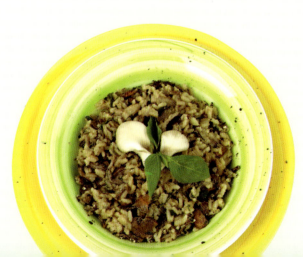

Preheat the oven to 190°C/375°F/gas mark 5. Dice the eggplant into 1 in. (2.5 cm) pieces and add, along with the other fresh vegetables, to a large ovenproof casserole dish. Pour over the canned tomatoes, vegetable stock, olive oil, and paprika and stir well. Cover the casserole dish and cook in the oven for 50-70 minutes.

desserts

strawberries with passion fruit sauce

Rich in betacarotene, and vitamin C.

Serves 4

1½ lb (700 g) small strawberries
12 oz (350 g) raspberries
1 passion fruit
2 tbsp honey

Place the raspberries and honey in a saucepan and gently heat to release the juices.

When the juices start to run, simmer for five minutes, stirring occasionally. Set aside and allow to cool.

Halve the passion fruit and, using a teaspoon, scoop out the seeds and juice into a small bowl.

Put the raspberries and passion fruit into a food processor and blend until smooth.

Place the raspberry and passion fruit sauce in a fine nylon sieve and press the purée through to remove the seeds.

Spoon out some of the sauce over the strawberries and serve.

fruit platter with spices

Rich in nutrients to provide an energy boost during a detox.

Serves 6

1 pineapple
2 papayas
1 small melon
juice of 2 limes
2 pomegranates
ground ginger
sprigs of mint

Peel the pineapple and remove the core and "eyes". Cut the flesh lengthways into thin wedges. Peel the papayas, cut them in half and then into thin wedges. Halve the melon and remove the seeds and once again cut into thin wedges with the skin removed.

Arrange the fruit on six individual plates and sprinkle with the lime juice. Cut the pomegranates in half, scoop out and scatter the seeds over the fruit. Sprinkle with a little ginger, and a few sprigs of mint. Serve immediately.

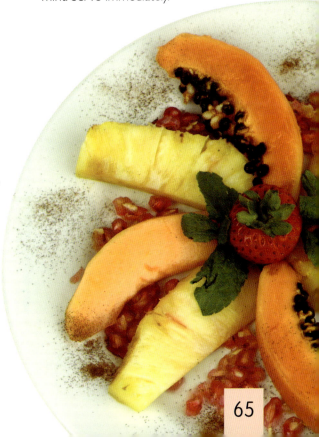

exercise

The benefits of exercise are widely recognized in all fields of medicine. It improves circulation and breathing, which benefits a detox program. It also reduces the risk of heart disease, high blood pressure, and high cholesterol.

Exercise does not necessarily mean spending hours at a time in the gym, "pumping iron". Most of the things we do throughout the day require energy to perform them. Simple things such as walking up and down stairs, vacuuming the house, gardening, and spring cleaning all require us to use our muscles, and get the heart beating a little faster, the blood flowing and our breathing increasing. Swimming is also good for fitness, as is walking, which we will look at later. We should all exercise in moderation to reap the health benefits. But if you are suffering from ill health you should always consult your doctor before embarking on any exercise program.

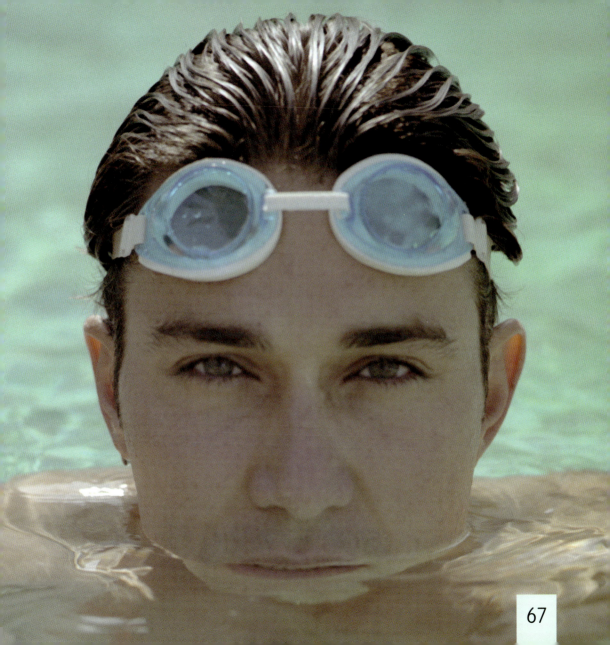

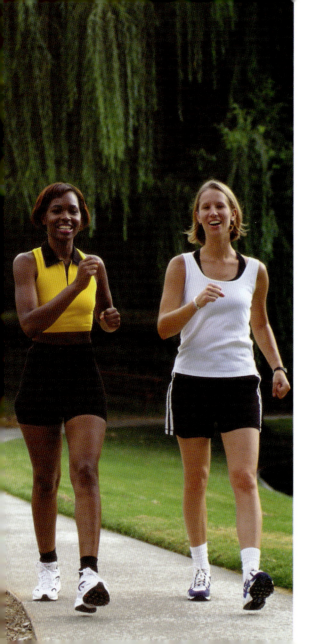

walking
and stretching

Have you ever watched a cat or a dog when they wake up? The first thing they do is stretch. We automatically stretch our limbs. It is something we do to help keep our muscles toned and stretched to their normal length. The reason for this is that usually when we wake we are about to embark on some form of physical activity, even if it is just walking downstairs to eat breakfast! It is our body's way of getting the muscles and joints ready for the activities ahead. Without stretching we are more prone to muscle strains.

Everyone would benefit from a stretch routine first thing in the morning. There are many ways to stretch, but the important thing is not to strain the muscles; remember stretching should feel good. Before starting, gently warm up, this can be through gentle movements such as walking on the spot and "rolling" our shoulders.

Once our bodies are warmed up and stretched we are prepared for physical activity. One of the best forms of exercise is walking—it's free, easy to do, and you don't need any special equipment! Walking helps to improve our circulation and lungs, it increases our heart rate, helps burn calories, and improves our fitness levels. Start off at a slow, steady pace and, as you get fitter, you may even start on those hill walks!

During a detox, walking helps us to remove toxins as the circulation is pumping blood through our body faster, we are sweating more, which removes toxins through the skin, and our breathing is increased, which removes toxins in the breath.

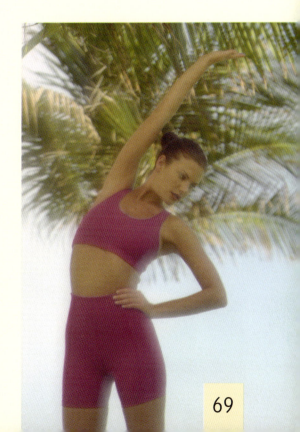

Why not explore alternative therapies and practices that can benefit the process of detox?

yoga

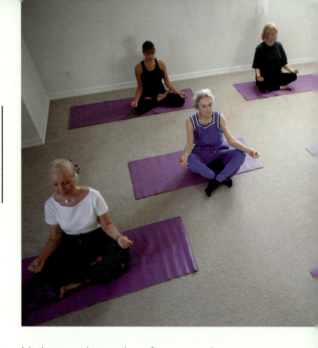

The popularity of yoga has increased in recent years and its health-giving benefits are supported by conventional and alternative health practitioners.

There are five main forms of yoga. Physical yoga is called Hatha yoga, and there are four mental yogas, Bhakti yoga for emotions, Gyana yoga for wisdom, Raja yoga for meditation, and Karma yoga for actions. For maximum benefit, these should all be practiced together, but people usually start with the Hatha yoga.

Hatha yoga is a series of postures that train and discipline the body and mind. It exercises the organs, nerves, and glands in the body, and also tones the muscles, which are gently stretched, creating greater flexibility. Circulation is improved and fat is eliminated, so it is a good way to control weight. It also teaches breath control, which is important for health, and also meditative postures to counteract a stressful lifestyle.

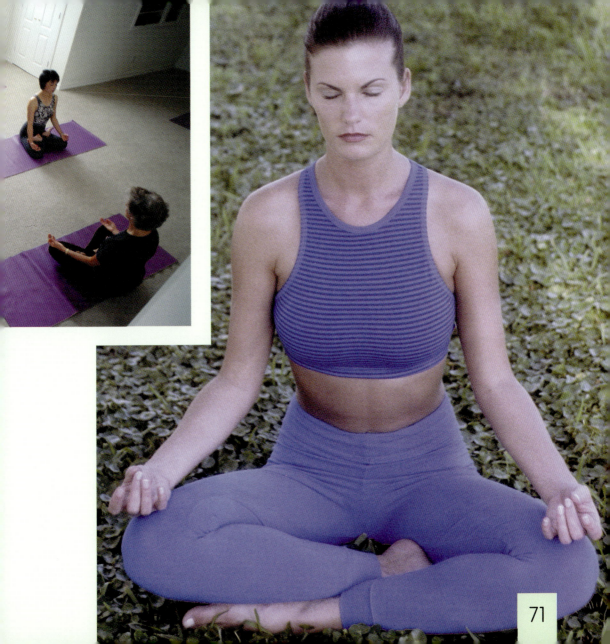

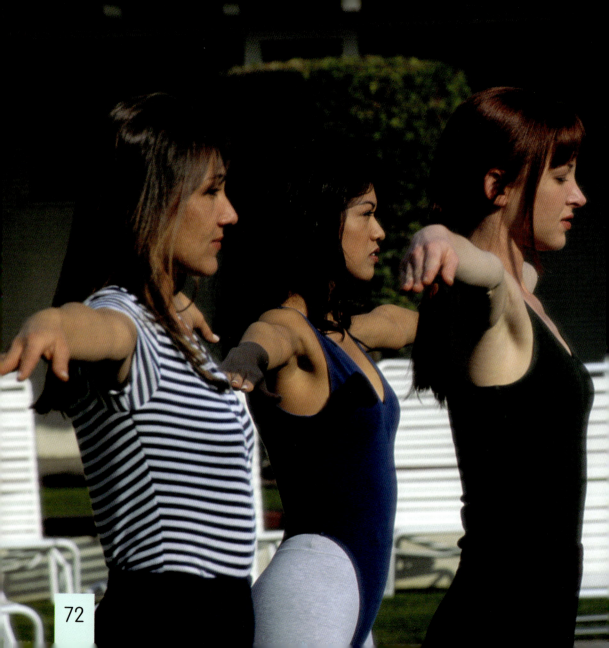

t'ai chi

T'ai chi is an ancient form of slow, gentle, rhythmic exercise, which originated in China. The movements of t'ai chi gently tone and strengthen the muscles and organs, improve circulation and posture, and relax both body and mind.

T'ai chi teaches patience and relaxation, and is a perfect antidote for the stress of modern lifestyles. It aims to restore balance to the body's systems and unblock the energy channels, but unlike acupressure and reflexology, it is practiced using gentle, relaxing movements.

T'ai chi is perfect for all ages. People with general joint aches and pains, even rheumatic and arthritic conditions, have benefited from this gentle form of exercise.

Regular detox sessions combined with a daily routine of t'ai chi work well together, with a more relaxed physical and mental state promoting the expulsion of toxins.

acupressure

Acupressure is the name given to the technique of stimulating the same points as those in acupuncture, but by using fingertip pressure rather than needles. It is used to treat most of the same conditions as acupuncture, and is ideal for people with a fear of needles.

Acupressure is similar to reflexology, in that it acts to unblock energy channels throughout the body. The difference is acupressure uses points across the whole body and not just those found on feet.

According to traditional Chinese medicine, there are 365 acupoints, or pressure points, throughout the body, and these run along the energy channels, or meridians.

When an acupoint is very tender from slight pressure, then it implies that there is a problem in the part of the body that is associated with that point.

Acupressure is a very gentle and relaxing therapy. It is ideal during a detox, as it will help to stimulate the body.

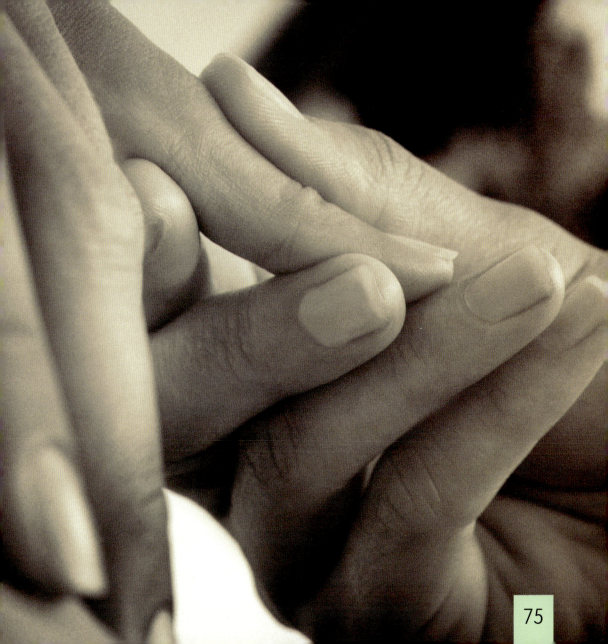

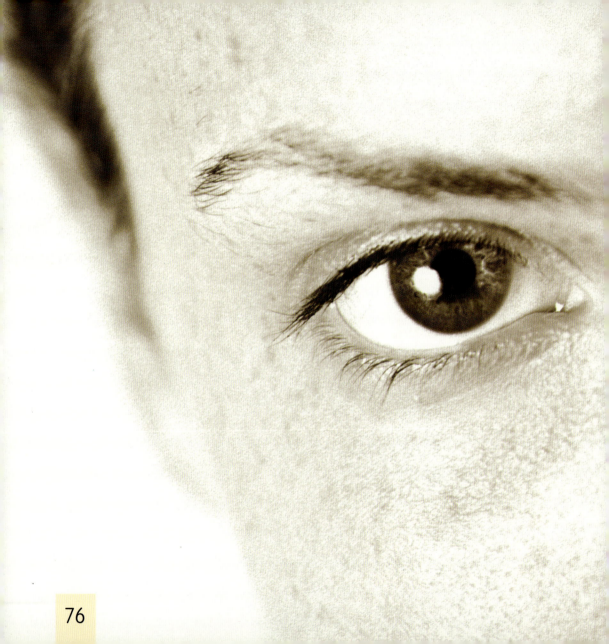

reiki

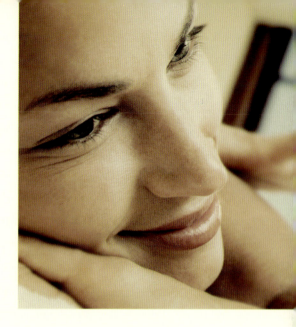

Reiki is a system of healing that can deal with problems of any kind, whether physical, emotional or mental. It often succeeds where other treatments have failed, and works to release accumulated daily stress, which is ideal for today's hectic, stressful lifestyles.

Reiki uses a hands-on technique that both relies upon and helps to develop strong instincts for where the treatments need to be directed on the body. It often gives the recipient a lift, while at the same time allowing them to relax.

This therapy can both heal the cause and eliminate the effect of the imbalance detected. It can be combined with other treatment methods, especially massage, aromatherapy, reflexology, or acupressure.

During a detox, reiki can help to alleviate some of the side effects that the program can bring, such as headaches, and can help boost the body's immune system.

reflexology

Reflexology is a form of foot massage originating in China around 5,000 years ago.

It is based on the principle that points on the feet correspond to organs and structures of the body, and are linked by energy channels or zones. When illness occurs, the corresponding channel becomes blocked.

Reflexology aims to destroy the blocks, allowing the energy to flow once again. It also helps to improve circulation and cleanse the body of harmful toxins.

We know that the body cleanses itself, mainly by using the lymphatic and excretory systems, but if these become blocked or do not function properly the toxins and waste products build up.

Reflexology will give a deep relaxation, helping all the bodily systems to function more efficiently, while at the same time unblocking the channels and creating a state where the body can once again eliminate waste products.

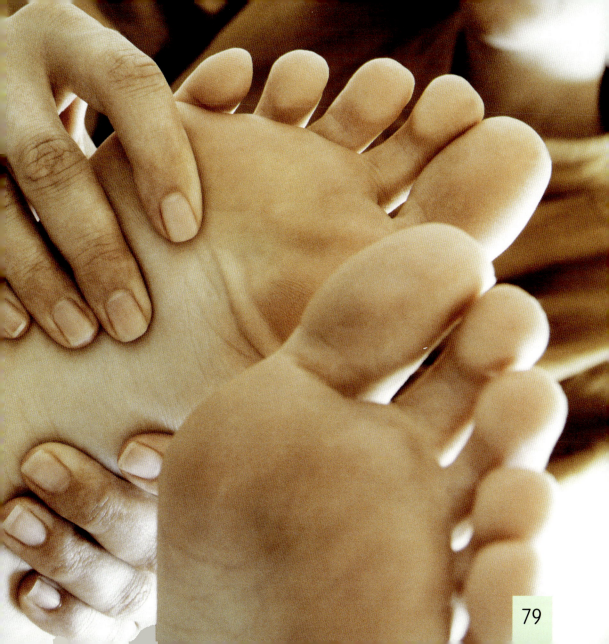

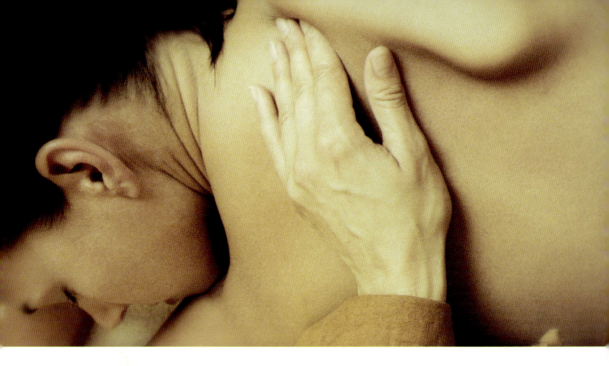

massage

The healing power of touch has been recognized for thousands of years.

It has been practiced for centuries, since the earliest civilizations, to heal, invigorate, and soothe the body. Even today we instinctively rub and massage the body if it is sore or aching.

The origin of the word "massage" lies both in the Arabian word "mass", which means "to press gently" and also the

Greek word "massage"—"to knead". Using fats and oils for lubrication body is referred to in the Bible and the Koran.

The earliest evidence of massage being practiced is found in the wall paintings of ancient cave dwellers which show people massaging each other.

In 3,000 BC the Chinese were practicing massage to cure ailments and improve health. The massage techniques spread to Japan where they were further developed. The practice of massage then spread into Europe, where it was well established by 500 BC.

Massage continued to be used to treat medical conditions until the 1960s in the UK, when the use of electrical-based equipment increased, and massage therapy was taken out of hospitals and used mainly in health farms and leisure centers. Today, massage in its various forms is being used once again to treat physical ailments, as well as for its relaxing and soothing effects.

One of the benefits of massage is its effect on both the circulatory and lymphatic systems, both of which are essential in the detox process. The circulatory system carries blood to all the organs, and the lymphatic system carries waste and toxins to the lymph nodes where it is filtered and passed into the bloodstream. If either of the systems are not functioning correctly then problems can occur. Massage helps to stimulate these systems.

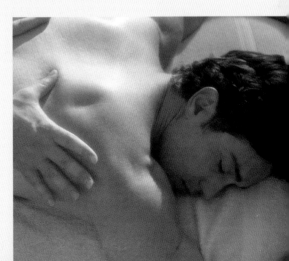

We do not have to seek the services of a therapist to benefit from a massage. There are many basic self-massage techniques that we can use.

There are a few things you need to remember before you start:

- don't massage over any skin infections, bruises, bumps, recently broken, or fractured bones, or varicose veins.
- always massage towards the heart.
- avoid massage if you have any history of embolism or thrombosis.

It is best if you sit on a towel on the floor and use small amounts of carrier oil which you can replenish regularly.

Begin with the feet and gently massage your soles and toes. Then take each leg in turn and, paying special attention to your calves, work upwards using firm, rhythmic strokes.

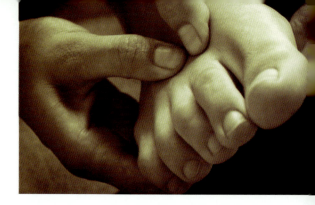

With one hand, gently knead your other hand. Use your thumb to firmly knead away the tension in your palm. You will be surprised how much tension is stored there.

Using your whole hand, gently stroke up the arm. Repeat on the other arm. Next, place your thumbs at either side of your spine at the base of your back, just above your pelvis. Using small, circular movement, gently work outwards, towards your sides. Repeat that about five times to loosen any tightness.

Using one hand, reach around towards the shoulder blade and firmly stroke back towards the chest. Repeat five times.

Next, with one arm, reach over your shoulder, and using your fingertips, firmly knead the muscles. This will be very tight as a lot of tension is stored there. Massage the whole area for about three minutes and then repeat on the other shoulder.

Using the tips of your fingers, start at the base of your neck, on either side of the vertebrae, and gently knead up towards the base of the skull. Repeat this five times.

Next, using the tips of your fingers and thumbs together, massage the whole of the scalp in small circular motions to relieve all the tension stored in the muscles there.

Finally, starting at the bridge of your nose, use two fingers and a circular motion, to work your way gently across your forehead to your temples. Finish with about one minute of massage there.

You should now be feeling very relaxed and most of the tension in your muscles will have been released. It is advisable to drink a large glass of water once you have finished, as this will help to get rid of the toxins and waste that have been flushed out of your muscles and cells.

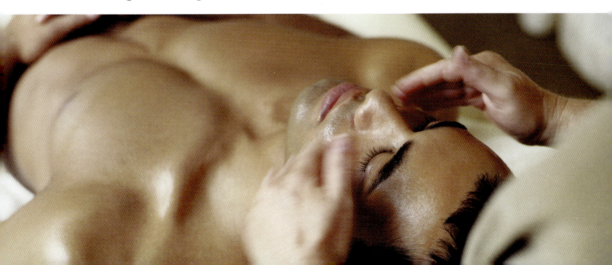

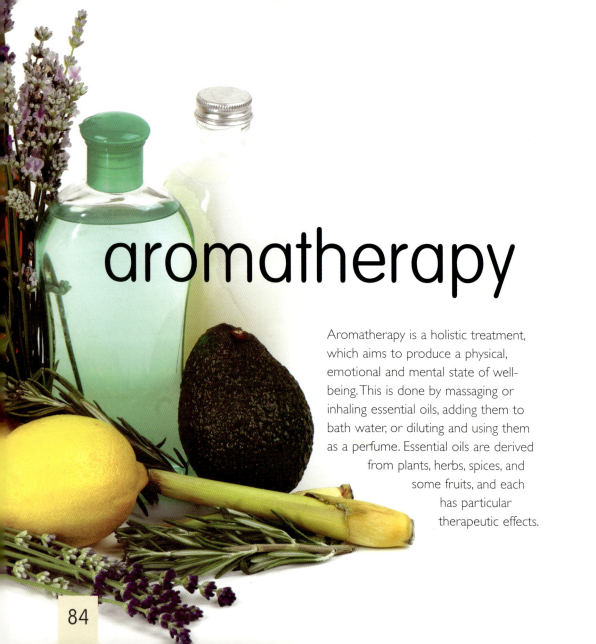

aromatherapy

Aromatherapy is a holistic treatment, which aims to produce a physical, emotional and mental state of well-being. This is done by massaging or inhaling essential oils, adding them to bath water, or diluting and using them as a perfume. Essential oils are derived from plants, herbs, spices, and some fruits, and each has particular therapeutic effects.

There are many essential oils, and with the exception of lavender and tea tree, they must not be applied directly to the skin without being diluted in a carrier oil, such as grapeseed oil. Essential oils should never be taken internally.

For use in massage, six drops should be added to four teaspoons of carrier oil. To use in the bath, add the same mixture to warm bath water. The oils can be vaporized in a bowl of hot water, or used in an oil burner. To use as a perfume, a few drops can be diluted in a small amount of alcoholic spirit, such as vodka, and dabbed onto the skin.

During a detox, aromatherapy can help you to relax and make the experience more pleasurable.

The following list describes the best detoxifying oils, their uses and also occasions when they should be avoided.

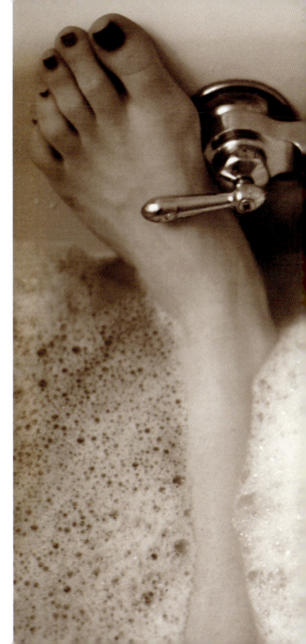

Essential oils are very concentrated and potent; if you are in any doubt about using them, always seek advice from a qualified aromatherapist.

lemon

As we have already seen, lemons have great detox qualities. Lemon oil is particularly good for purifying the liver, digestive problems and as a cardiac stimulant. You should avoid the sun or sunbeds for 6-8 hours after use, and it can irritate sensitive skin.

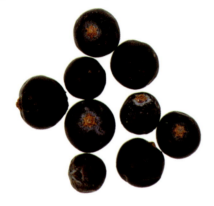

juniper berry

This is probably the most detoxifying of the essential oils. It is used for liver problems, purification, urinary infections and as a diuretic. It should not be used during pregnancy or if suffering from kidney problems. Mixed with rosemary and used in the bath, it is an excellent hangover remedy.

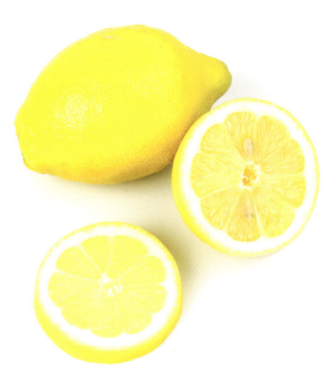

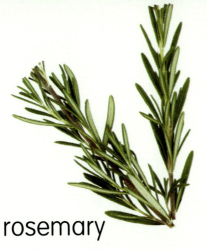

tea tree

One of the most powerful antiseptics, yet gentle on the skin, tea tree has been added here for its immunity-boosting properties. It is safe to use on all but the most sensitive of skins and will help with colds, flu, fungal, viral, and bacterial infections.

rosemary

This oil is a good liver decongestant, it improves circulation, is good for intestinal upsets and also for fluid retention. However, it should not be used during pregnancy, or by people suffering from epilepsy.

lavender

Lavender oil is safe to use undiluted on the skin, it is also excellent for stress, respiratory problems and general well-being. During a detox this oil can help to keep you in good cheer.

face masks

Our faces are in constant contact with pollutants. The following face masks are made with natural ingredients and the herbal decoctions can be purchased from most health food stores.

To prepare them, mix the ingredients together in a bowl. Once mixed, spread over the whole of the face, avoiding the eyes and mouth. Leave on for ten minutes, rinse off with warm water and pat the face dry.

moisturizing masks

Recipe:
3 tbsp mashed fresh avocado
1 tbsp ground dried orange peel
3 tbsp marsh mallow root decoction
3 tbsp warmed honey

Recipe:
3 tbsp grated fresh apples with peel
3 tbsp mashed fresh peaches
3 tbsp dandelion root decoction
2 tbsp organic milk or goat's milk

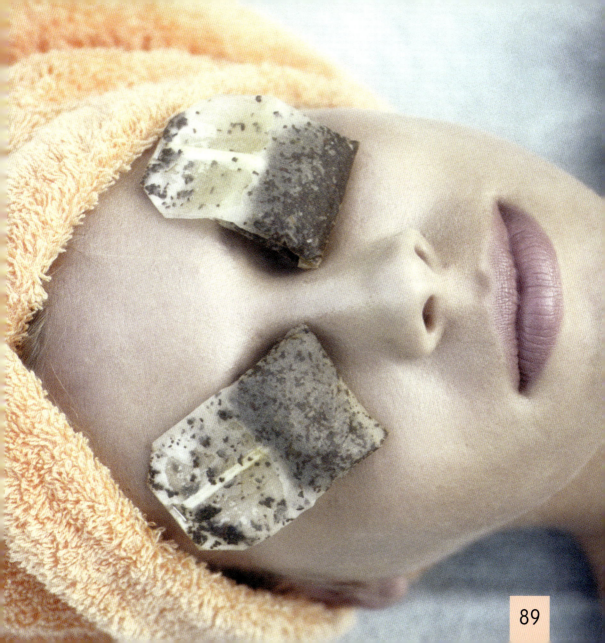

nourishing and toning masks

Recipe:
2 tbsp ground almonds
2 tbsp mashed banana
3 tbsp rosewater
2 tbsp warmed honey
2 tbsp organic milk or goat's milk

Recipe:
4 tbsp mashed cooked carrots
2 tbsp parsley infusion
2 tbsp warmed honey
2 tbsp comfrey leaf

Recipe:
2 tbsp fresh mashed strawberry
2 tbsp natural yogurt
3 tbsp fresh mashed avocado
2 tbsp calendula flower infusion

Recipe:
3 tbsp ground kelp (grind in a clean coffee grinder!)
2 tbsp comfrey root decoction
3 tbsp mashed cooked celery
1 beaten egg white

Recipe:
4 tbsp mashed fresh papaya
2 tbsp warmed honey
6 fresh grapes mashed or puréed
2 tbsp bay leaf infusion
3 tbsp buttermilk

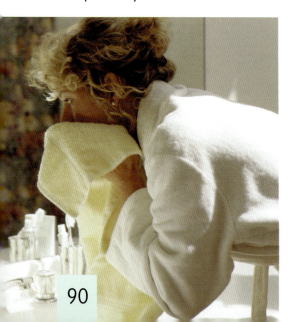

to combat oily skin

Recipe:
3 tbsp mashed fresh apricot
2 tbsp freshly squeezed lemon juice
3 tbsp natural yogurt
1 beaten egg white

Recipe:
4 tbsp peeled and mashed cucumber
3 tbsp ground almonds
1 tbsp witch hazel tincture
2 tbsp organic milk or goat's milk

sensitive or irritated skin

Recipe:
3 tbsp comfrey root decoction
3 tbsp mashed fresh avocado
2 tbsp buttermilk
2 tbsp rosewater
1 tbsp finely ground almonds

Patch test: Those with sensitive skin should test these recipes first. Apply a small amount to the inside of your wrist, leave for 24 hours, do not use if irratation occurs.

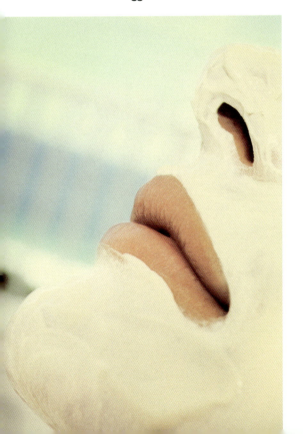

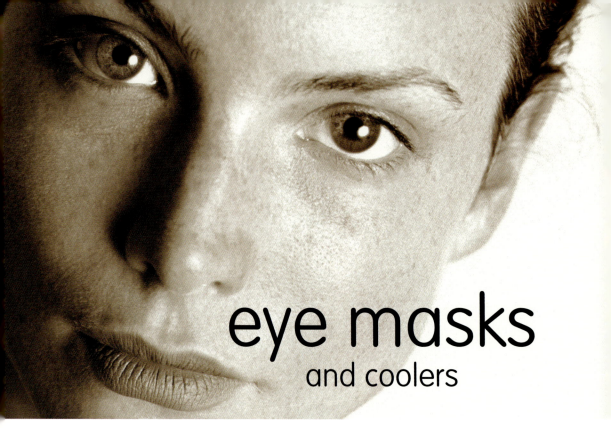

eye masks
and coolers

Your eyes are hard-working organs, and are subject to a lot of strain and pollution. They are bombarded with dust and UV rays on a daily basis. We need to care for them just as much as we care for the rest of our body.

Eye masks are perfect for soothing them. Placed in the fridge so they reach a pleasant cooling temperature, they reduce redness and puffiness, and help to ease the tension around the eyes. Alternatively you can use a slice of cool cucumber on each eye, or used, cold tea bags. This aloe eye balm will also refresh tired eyes.

aloe under-eye balm

This easy under-eye pick-me-up can be left on overnight to help rejuvenate tired eyes, and keeps fairly well if put in a sealed glass, wide-mouthed jar. Remember that anything you put near the eye area can get into the eyes, so be very careful and those with sensitive skin should do a patch test first.

1½ tsp wheat germ oil
½ tsp vitamin E oil
1 tsp aloe gel
1 tsp honey (for vegans omit honey and increase aloe by ½ tsp and wheat germ by ½ tsp)
1½ tsp cocoa butter
5 drops calendula essential oil

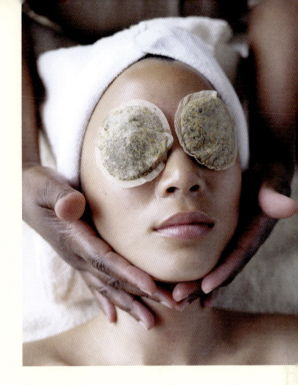

First, melt the cocoa butter in a pan with the wheat germ oil and vitamin E. Remove from heat and beat in the aloe and honey, if you are including honey in your preparation. Add the calendula essential oil at the end once the other ingredients are well blended. Pour it into a small pot and apply sparingly UNDER the eye area only as needed.

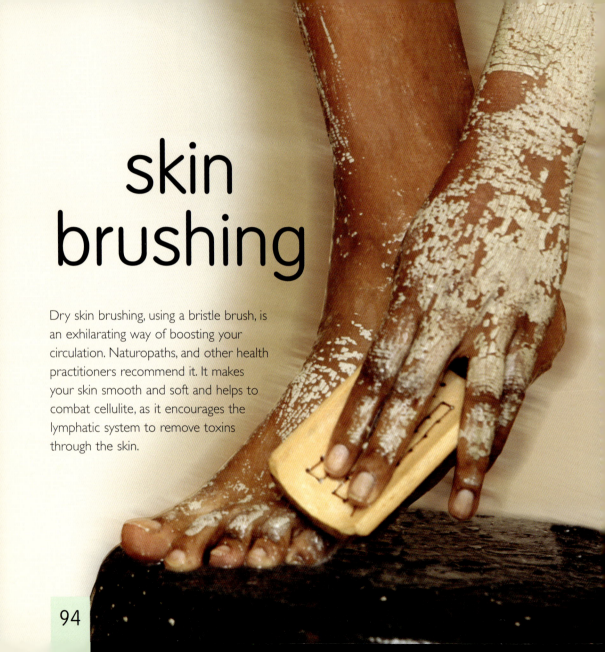

skin brushing

Dry skin brushing, using a bristle brush, is an exhilarating way of boosting your circulation. Naturopaths, and other health practitioners recommend it. It makes your skin smooth and soft and helps to combat cellulite, as it encourages the lymphatic system to remove toxins through the skin.

Skin brushing the whole body should take around ten minutes and ideally should be done before a bath or shower. If done before an aromatherapy bath, it makes it easier for the essential oils to penetrate the skin.

Starting at your feet and toes, brush up the front and back of your legs using long strokes. As in massage, the strokes should always be done towards the heart.

Move up your thighs and then brush over your buttocks, and up to your lower back.

Brush your arms and hands, stroking towards the heart, again using long, slow strokes.

Skin brushing should not be confined to when you are on a detox program. You should include it in your daily routine, as it will exfoliate and rejuvenate your skin, and improve circulation and lymph drainage. Try it for a week and see the difference.

Brush your stomach to stimulate the colon. You should use circular, clockwise movements. Move across your shoulders, down over your chest, then down your back.

Never brush your face and use only a dry brush on your body. The pressure you use depends on the strength of your skin, so use light, slow pressure at first and increase the pressure with each session as your skin becomes stronger.

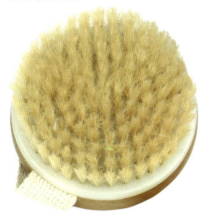

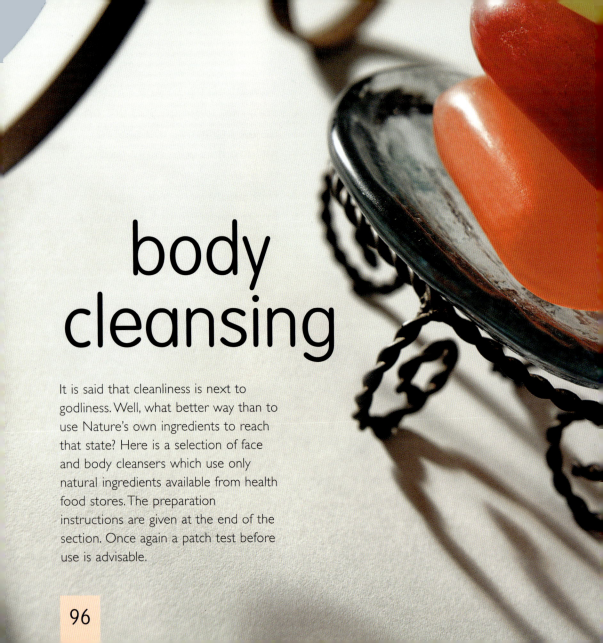

body cleansing

It is said that cleanliness is next to godliness. Well, what better way than to use Nature's own ingredients to reach that state? Here is a selection of face and body cleansers which use only natural ingredients available from health food stores. The preparation instructions are given at the end of the section. Once again a patch test before use is advisable.

good general purpose cleanser

3 part whole oats
3 part organic dried milk or goat's milk
2 part lavender flowers
2 part comfrey root

Suggestions: add two drops lavender oil to every 4 oz (115 g) of dry recipe, mix together, and store. For washing, use water, milk, or green tea.

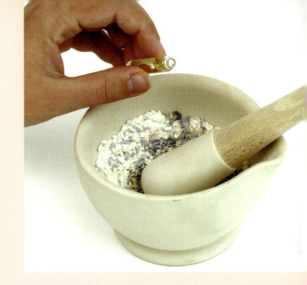

to cleanse and exfoliate

3 part whole oats
3 part organic dried milk or goat's milk
1 part sea salt
1 part rosemary
1 part orange peel

Suggestions: add two drops of rosemary or orange oil to every 4 oz (115 g) of dry recipe, mix and bottle. For washing, use water, milk, or herbal tea.

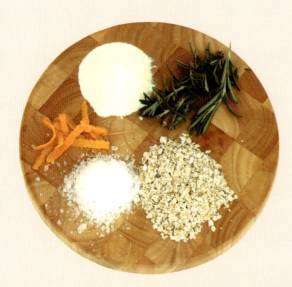

to cleanse and moisturize

3 part whole oats
3 part organic dried milk or goat's milk
1 part camomile flowers
1 part calendula flowers
1 part slippery elm bark

Suggestions: for washing, use water, milk, or warmed honey.

Warning: Slippery elm bark should not be used while pregnant.

to cleanse and combat oily skin

3 part whole oats
1 part fullers earth or kaolin clay
1 part brewers yeast
1 part grapefruit or lemon peel
2 part calendula flowers
2 part peppermint leaves

Suggestions: add two drops peppermint or grapefruit oil to every 4 oz (115 g). For washing, use water, witch hazel, or green tea.

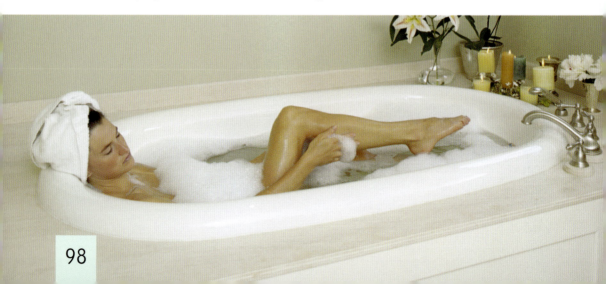

to nourish and clarify skin

2 part whole oats
3 part organic dried milk or goat's milk
1 part sage leaves
2 part lavender flowers
1 part kelp
1 part green clay

Suggestions: add two drops rose or geranium oil to every 4 oz (115 g) of dry mixture and bottle. For washing, use water, milk, or nettle tea.

easy exfoliator

1 part whole oats
1 part almonds
1 part lavender flower
1 part powdered milk

Suggestions: add a few drops lavender oil. Store in a glass jar or ceramic container with a lid.

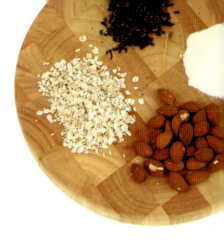

preparation instructions

Grind all ingredients individually, either in a grinder, processor or by hand, and then blend in the proportions given. Once blended, you may add the essential oils as suggested, and store the mixture in a glass or ceramic container with a lid. Liquid is added per usage at the time you are actually washing yourself. You may use plain water, or combine it with the liquid suggestions given. You can make cleansers up ahead of time and if kept sealed in a cool dry spot, they will stay fresh for about six months. If kept in the refrigerator they will last almost indefinitely.

detox your mind

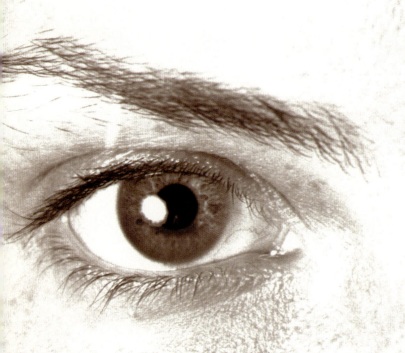

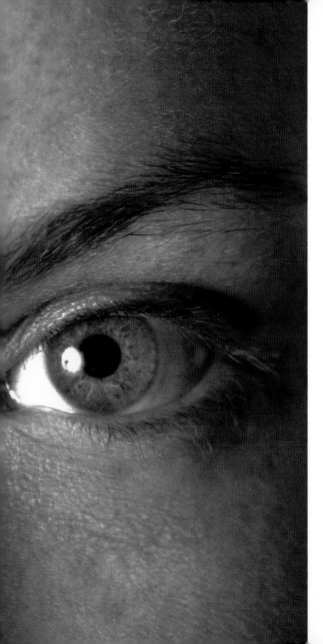

Have you ever tried to diet, but as soon as you become fed up or stressed, you turned back to junk food? As the old saying goes, "A healthy body needs a healthy mind". This is certainly true with diets and also with detoxing. As you follow a detox program, you may suffer some side effects, and so a positive mental attitude is needed.

Relaxed breathing techniques or meditation can help to sustain the right frame of mind.

Detoxing itself will help us to gain mental clarity and to feel more relaxed and revitalized. This will help us achieve better quality rest. Once we have this it will make us feel more like sticking to a healthier lifestyle and keeping to some sort of detox program.

In this section we will look at meditation and techniques that can be used in our everyday lives.

meditation

Meditation calms the mind and nervous system and lowers the heart rate. The rhythm of the breath slows down considerably and this slowing down enables us to cope with pressure increases. Meditation enhances sensitivity, alertness and mental clarity.

Meditation is best practiced at the beginning and end of the day. Practice for fifteen minutes to an hour, in a quiet space, either indoors or out. Keep the spine straight and the body still; choose a well-backed chair, or a cushion placed on the floor. Rest your hands on your thighs with your thumbs and forefingers touching, or join them across your abdomen.

This breathing technique will help to release any surplus tensions and toxicity from the lungs. Inhale slowly and deeply through the nose and hold the breath in the abdomen for six seconds.

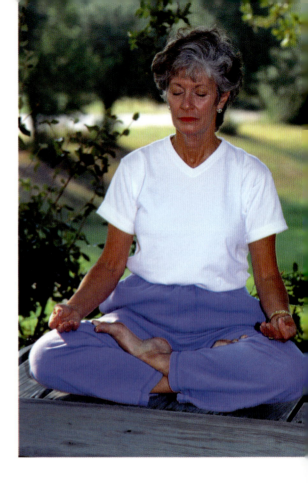

Purse the lips and exhale a little breath at a time through the mouth. Pause between each short exhalation for about a second until you have completely exhaled, and then pause for five seconds.

Repeat about six times.

This next exercise focusses the attention on the natural flow of the breath as it travels through the nose into the body and out again.

Sit in your chosen spot. Close your eyes softly.

Begin to be aware of either the sensation of the breath as it touches the nostrils as you breathe in and out, or the rising and falling of your abdomen as you inhale and exhale.

Mentally follow the internal journey of the breath, as this will help focus the mind.

As the abdomen rises with inhalation, say to yourself "rising". As the abdomen falls with the exhalation, say "falling".

Keep the mind open and aware of the sensation, while continually repeating these words. It is important that the word corresponds with the sensation of the breath; otherwise it will become mechanical and meaningless.

The breath may be fast or slow. Try not to judge it or control it. Just observe it. Let it lead your attention. You are following the breath, not the breath following you.

Another form of meditation can be practiced through "visualization".

Picture yourself in a pleasant setting, such as on a beach surrounded by the ocean. Let yourself walk barefoot through the sand.

Use the strength of the breeze, the sound of the sea gulls, and the lap of the waves to evoke the scene. Let yourself be there, and totally relax.

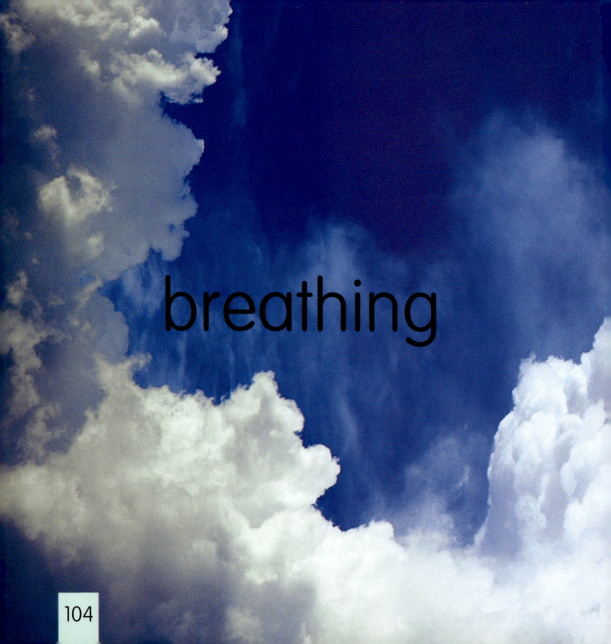

One of our most important functions is breathing, but the majority of us don't do it properly. If we are breathing correctly, the lower part of our stomach should rise first, followed by our chest, as we inhale and exhale slowly through the nose.

The following is a relaxation technique, which takes fifteen to twenty minutes to complete. It can be done sitting on a chair, lying on the floor, or in bed. It should be done in a quiet environment, and shoes should be removed. Use the same pattern of breathing throughout. By the end of it, see how relaxed you are!

- take a deep breath in and point your toes. Hold for a count of six and exhale, letting out any tensions, let your feet open and relax.

- take a deep breath in and flex your feet up, pressing the calf muscles into the floor, hold for six and exhale. Release the legs.

- take a deep breath and pull up the muscles above the kneecap into the thighs and briefly hold; release the muscles and breath and let your thighs roll open.

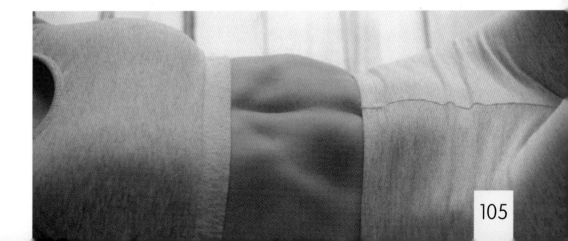

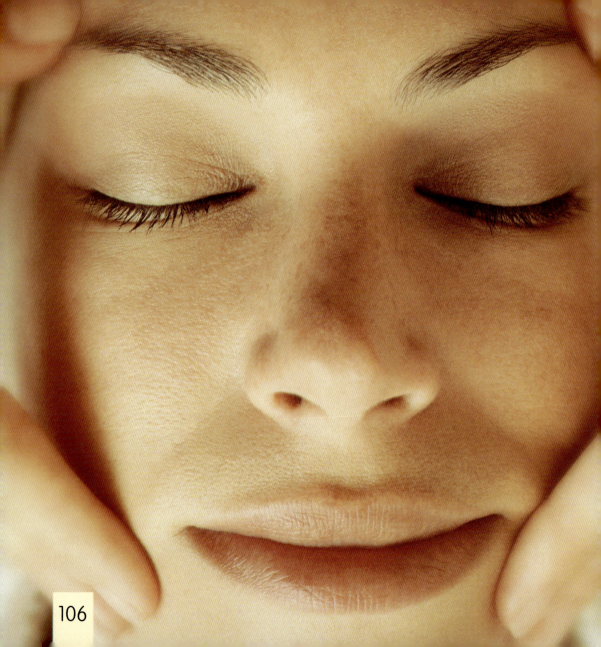

- take a deep breath in and squeeze your buttocks and abdomen tightly in. Release the muscles as you exhale.

- take a deep breath into the abdomen, then let it balloon out. Hold for a count of four. Exhale and relax.

- bend your elbows and make a fist. Breathe in and squeeze the deltoid muscles at the top of your arms. Exhale and release your arms.

- take a breath in and raise your shoulders to your ears, holding for a count of six. Exhale and relax your shoulders.

- as you breathe in, bring your palms in front of your chest and press them against each other. Hold and relax your arms.

- breathe in and expand your lungs and upper chest. Hold for a count of four and exhale.

- breathe in, raise your head from the floor and hold. Gently let it return to the floor as you exhale. If you are in a chair, slowly roll the head from side to side as you inhale and exhale.

- take a breath in and raise the eyebrows. Exhale and relax.

- breathe in and squeeze your face tight. Hold for a count of four and relax.

- breathe in and open your jaw wide. Hold for a count of four and exhale.

- take a deep breath into the chest and hold. Release just half of it, then take another breath into the abdomen and hold. Exhale it slowly.

Your body should now be totally relaxed and all your cells filled with life-giving oxygen.

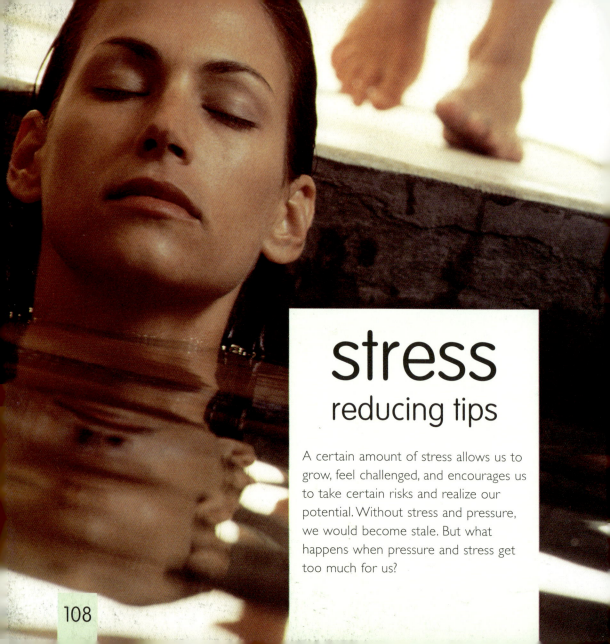

stress
reducing tips

A certain amount of stress allows us to grow, feel challenged, and encourages us to take certain risks and realize our potential. Without stress and pressure, we would become stale. But what happens when pressure and stress get too much for us?

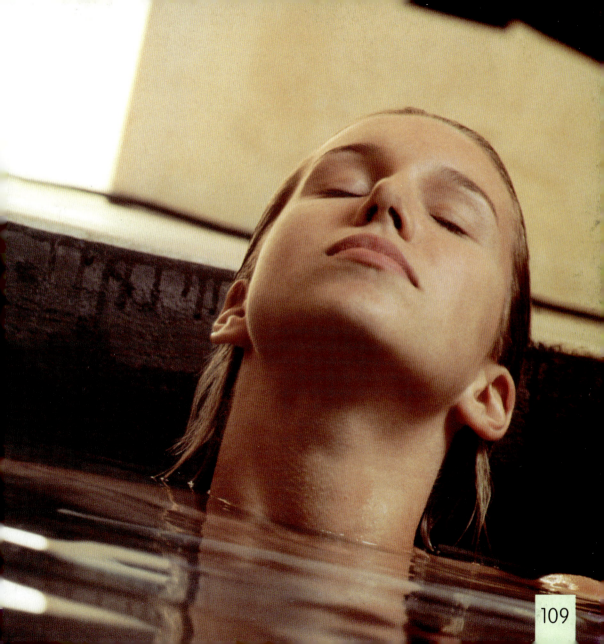

There are many stress-related disorders; here are just some of them:

- palpitations
- shortness of breath
- insomnia
- hair loss
- indigestion, irritable bowel syndrome and digestive problems
- migraines and headaches
- lethargy
- being overtired and depressed

To help reduce the amount of negative stress we face daily, we need balance in the four main areas of our lives.

home environment

Home should be our sanctuary, somewhere where there is a certain order and peace. We should feel nurtured here, emotionally, physically, and mentally. This is a place where our treasured possessions are safe and looked after. Our home is the place where we work out our deepest pressures and stress-related symptoms.

If things go wrong in this environment, and it becomes a place filled with anger and frustration, then it is important to seek a balance to the situation. The best method, for more serious problems, is to seek counseling. Talking through things with someone who is skilled in listening and advising is an effective way of dealing with stress in your life.

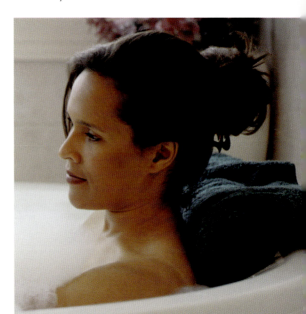

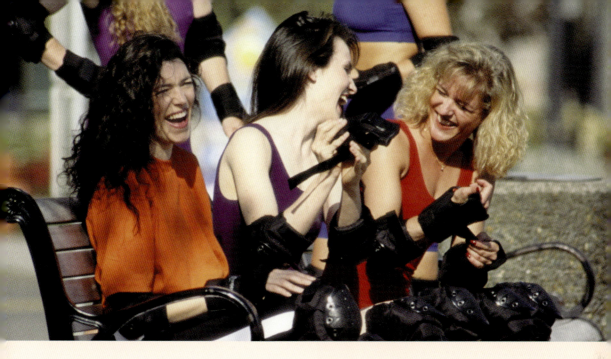

work

This is a place where our greatest challenges, and often our greatest achievements and fulfillments, happen. Our work is an arena in which we express all our greatest aspirations.

If you feel unfulfilled at work, then you should find ways to adjust the work you do so that it facilitates your aspirations in a more dynamic way. Do this by communicating with your bosses and colleagues.

friends

In a balanced lifestyle, it is important to have friends with whom you can share your feelings and relax completely.

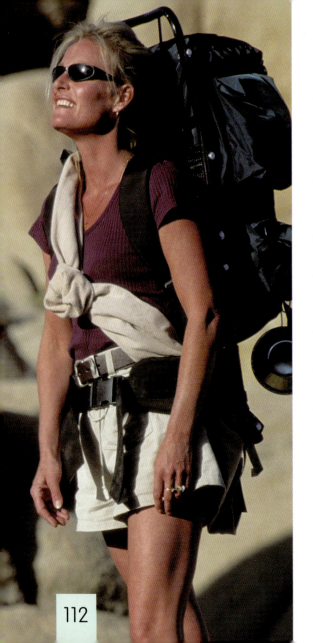

creative play

This is the way we relax ourselves through hobbies and leisure activities.

Going for walks, listening to music, watching a baseball match; it is whatever we do to take a break from our normal routine, to switch off from life and enjoy the moment. Here we can recharge, ready for the pressures of another day.

There are other ways to reduce stress in our lives. Healthy eating is one way. Eating the wrong foods can increase stress on our body, so it is important to have a balanced and nutritious diet. Exercise helps to rid our bodies of stress. Try swimming, joining a gym or attending a fitness class. If you don't enjoy such activities, then go walking, or cycling. Even if you just get off the bus one stop earlier, or walk to the shops instead of taking the car, it will help you to maintain a good level of fitness.

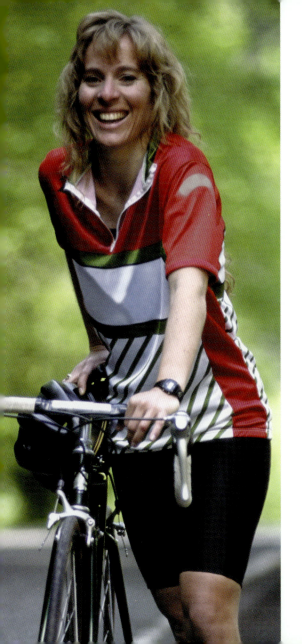

Regular holistic treatments, such as massage, aromatherapy, reflexology, and reiki can help reduce stress levels. Try giving your partner a massage, and get them to return the favor. You can even use the self-massage routine, found on page 82.

Take some time out to meditate, or practice the breathing technique, to help balance your mind and body.

One important thing is not to let stress get the better of you. It has a place in your life, but keep it where it belongs, under control, and do not let it grow and take over.

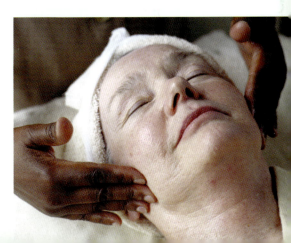

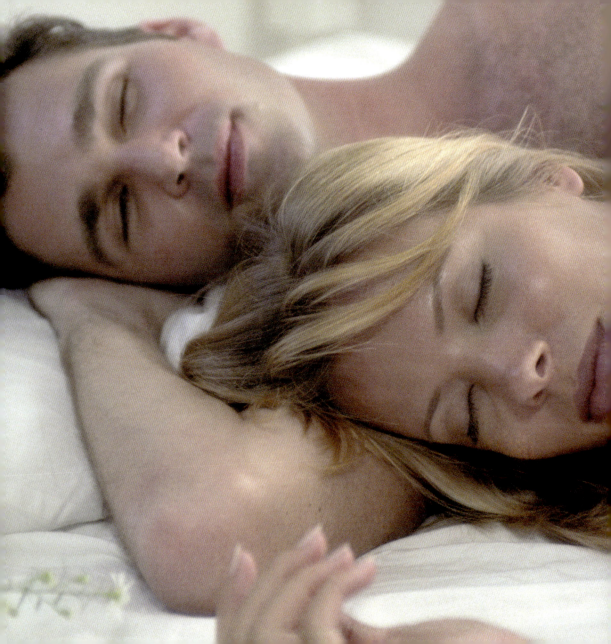

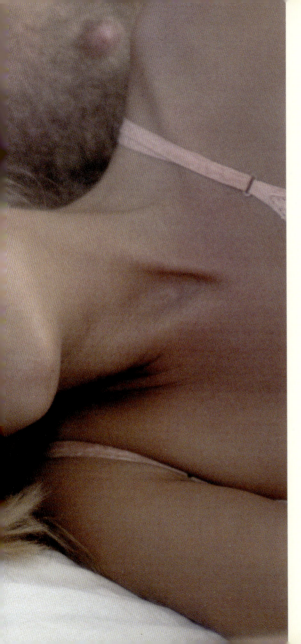

sleep

Human beings spend almost one third of their lives sleeping. It is the most natural and instinctive remedy to balance and replenish the energy that we use every day. It is also the time when our bodies work to regenerate our cells, tissues, and organs.

As we grow older, the amount of sleep we require diminishes. Babies need sixteen hours of sleep per day. With adults, this reduces to about six to eight.

Research has found that sleeping for less than four hours and more than eight can lead to reduced longevity. So you should aim for the recommended six to eight hours of sound sleep per night.

Don't underestimate the importance of good sleep. During a detox, when all the harmful wastes are being removed from your body, sleep helps to repair all the damage made by toxins.

There has been a lot of research on sleep, and one of the things we now know is that there are two types of sleep patterns, "orthodox" and "paradoxical".

Orthodox sleep has been divided into four separate levels of brain activity. The first being very light sleep, from which we can be easily woken, is when relaxation starts.

The second and third states are more relaxed. The muscles relax more deeply and the heart rate and breathing continue to slow down. The fourth level is a state of very deep sleep, the "delta" state.

Due to the increasingly rapid cell division which occurs, orthodox sleep is highly beneficial. This provides the body with the opportunity to renew and replenish itself. Growth hormones are also released into the blood stream in our deepest sleep state.

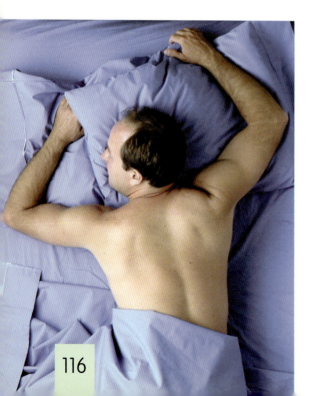

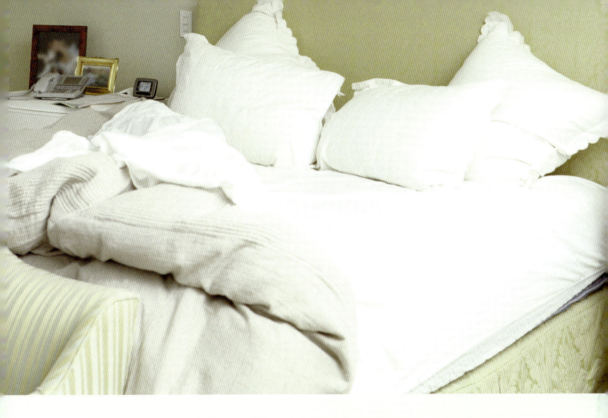

Paradoxical sleep is our mysterious dream state, when our brain waves begin to move more rapidly and irregularly than when we are awake. This helps to restore mental harmony. Other signs of increased heart rate and physical movements indicate that there is activity occurring on other levels of awareness—rapid eye movement (REM) is one such activity.

People who wake sporadically during a night's sleep will often feel tired, drowsy and dozy the next day because the ninety-

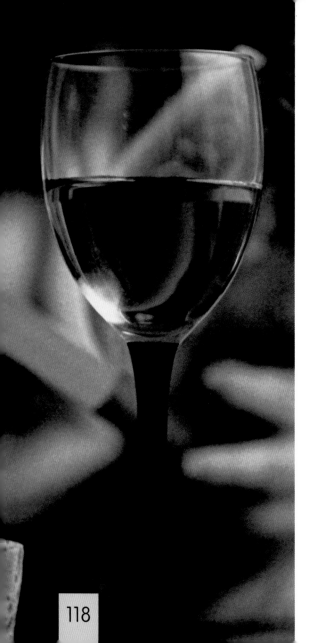

minute cycle of deep sleep and inner mental activity (paradoxical and orthodox sleep) is broken. There are many ways to improve sleep without turning to sleeping pills. If you do suffer from sleepless nights, try some of the following :

- exercise during the day often helps to make you tired at bedtime, but try not to exercise too late in the evening as the adrenaline rushing around your body will keep you awake.

- avoid caffeine in the evening.

- avoid alcohol.

- avoid heavy meals after 8 o'clock.

- use some of the breathing and relaxation techniques found earlier in this book.

- run cold water on your wrists if you cannot get to sleep.

- a few drops of lavender oil on your pillow may help (but only if you like the scent).

- the herbal remedy passiflora is a good sedative, and is safe and non-addictive.

- have a warm bath before bedtime. Add some of your favorite-smelling essential oils and turn it into an aromatherapy bath. The best ones to use are lavender, camomile, patchouli, sandalwood, and ylang ylang.

- camomile tea is very relaxing. This can be drunk in the evening to promote good sleep.

- don't lie in bed worrying about not being able to sleep as this usually makes sleep even more difficult. Instead, get up and walk around the house, read a book or listen to some relaxing music.

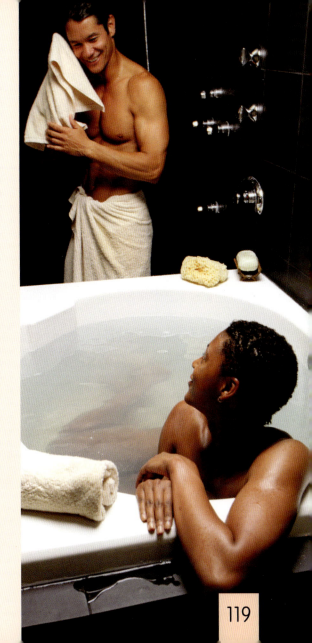

health spa treatments

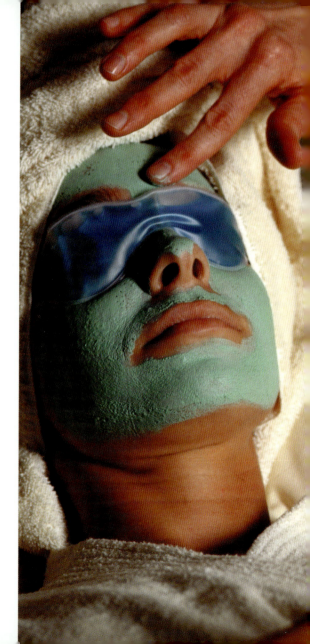

A day at a health spa is a very luxurious treat, and one that can be beneficial to both body and mind. What better way to reward yourself for completing the detox program than with a day being pampered by someone else?

As well as the usual massage treatments, jacuzzis and sauna, there are many different treatments that are ideal detoxifiers. The following are some of the more popular available at most good health spas.

body polish

A special blend of sea salts and essential oils is used in this full body exfoliation treatment. The salts and oils work together to soothe sore, aching muscles, open pores, and increase circulation, leaving your skin silky smooth.

dead sea mud mask

This detoxifying body wrap begins with a dry body brush followed by an aromatherapy steam bath. The warm mud is evenly applied over the entire surface of the body. The recipient is then wrapped for thirty minutes while the impurities are drawn out of the skin and the body's natural mineral supply is replenished. This treatment should end with the application of a light moisturizer.

marine powder wrap

This blend of sea algae, clay, and sea salts provides a vigorous detoxifying action that nourishes and tones all skin types and is excellent for those in a cellulite and weight loss program. The treatment should also include a dry body brush and moisturizer.

herbal cleansing facial

Only natural plant, earth, fruit, and herb extracts are used in this extremely relaxing facial treatment. This treatment includes: a deep cleansing, exfoliation; face, neck, and shoulder massage; and a herbal clay mask. While you relax, your arms, hands, and feet will be massaged. A special toner and moisturizer is then applied, leaving you feeling wonderful!

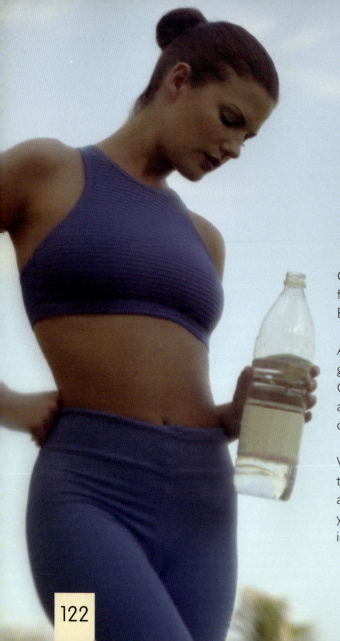

daily detox

Ok, you have completed your detox, for a day, a weekend, or even a week. But what now?

Are you going to go and undo all the great things you have just achieved? Chances are you will feel so good about yourself that you will want to carry on.

While it is often unwise to follow all these processes on a daily basis, there are a number of things you can add to your everyday life to keep your body in good health.

- drink at least eight glasses of water a day.

- cut out, or at least cut down on, the amount of tea, coffee, cola, and other sugary, fizzy drinks you drink. Opt for fruit juices and herbal teas instead.

- eat plenty of fresh fruit and vegetables, go organic if you can, and if not, thoroughly wash everything. Eat at least five different portions per day.

- cut down on dairy products and red meat.

- don't fry your food. This can increase the carcinogen in food. Instead, bake, boil or broil.

- each morning have a glass of warm water with some freshly squeezed lemon juice.

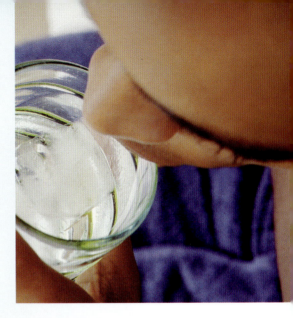

- skin brush each day. If you do not have the time to do it daily, use a loofah in the shower, to help exfoliate and clear away toxins.

- cut down on alcohol. If you can avoid it altogether then do so.

- do some gentle stretching exercises each morning.

- cut out all junk food.

- breathe properly. Try to learn the techniques in this book.

- buy a book on t'ai chi or yoga and learn some of the moves. Perform these daily to help your posture and keep you supple and flexible, relaxed and focussed.

- take a few minutes out of your day to sit in a quiet room to meditate, or at least just shut your eyes and relax. If you have a quiet place at work, just go and sit and calm your body and mind.

- Drink a cup of soothing camomile tea an hour before bedtime to help you to sleep. A warm bath with some essential oils will also help you sleep soundly.

If you can follow this on a daily basis, then the next time you start a detox, it will be easier, and side effects will be less in both number and severity.

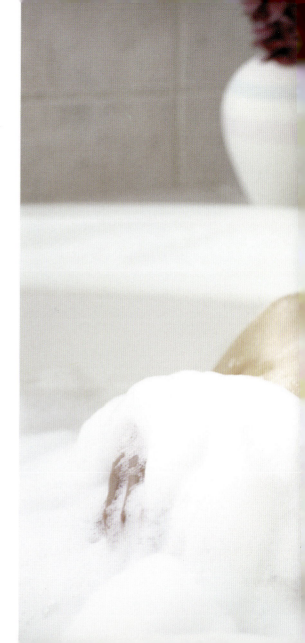

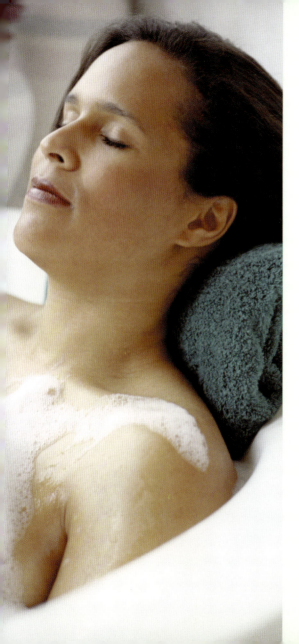

For one day each week you could eat just raw fruit, vegetables and fruit juice, and drink just water and herbal teas. This will give your body another chance to repair and renew itself.

The results of all these efforts will not go unnoticed. You will notice an improvement in your skin, hair, and eyes. You will have lots of energy, less negative stress, and you will feel alive!

The long-term effects can be even better. You should find you have fewer colds and infections. Your stress levels should be reduced, because you are dealing with problems more effectively and positively. Your health may improve and any aches and pains should lessen. A healthier body through detox should also be less susceptible to chronic conditions such as cancer, high blood pressure, and arthritis.

For such small and easy changes to your life, the rewards are many and great.

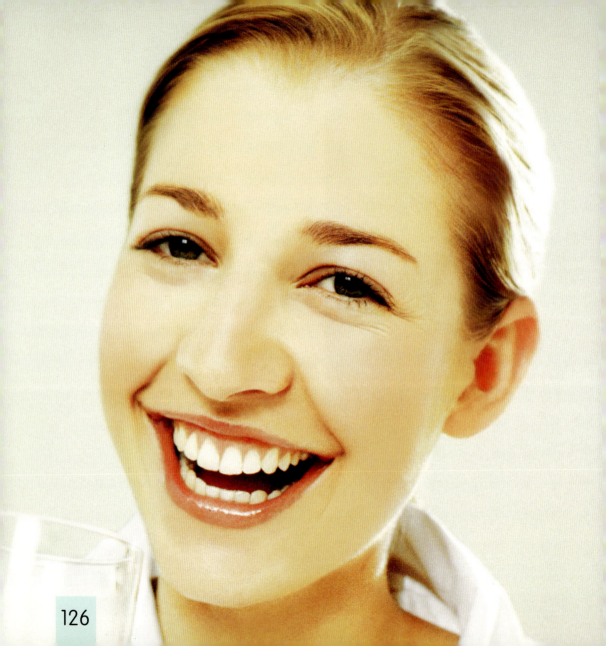

glossary

antioxidants
Chemicals that are capable of detoxifying the harmful "free radicals" or oxidants in our systems which can trigger cancer, arterial damage, inflammation and aging.

betacarotene
An antioxidant. This is a yellowish pigment in vegetables that is converted in the body to vitamin A.

blueberry extract
An antioxidant, available as a liquid from health food stores.

biotin
A B-complex vitamin.

carcinogen
Any substance likely to cause cancer.

free radicals
These are atoms or molecules in the body that have become charged. They roam the body in great numbers, damaging normal cells.

lipoic acid
An antioxidant that is found in yeast.

lymphatic system
The system in our bodies that is responsible for producing our immunity-boosting cells and removing waste fluids and toxins.

milk thistle
This herbal extract can be purchased from health food stores. It is a good detoxifier and helps to protect the liver.

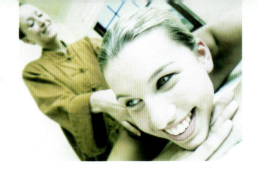

minerals

These are essential for good health, and can be found in fresh foods.

probiotics

Beneficial bacteria, found naturally in the gut. Destroyed by antibiotics, they can be found in natural yogurt, and purchased in tablet form at health food stores.

reiki

A very relaxing healing process which uses a hands-on technique.

selenium

A mineral, with antioxidant properties. Found in seafood. Supplements are needed if you are vegetarian.

vitamins

Found in fresh foods, these are organic substances needed by the body in small amounts, for survival.

- vitamin A can be found in carrots, dark green vegetables, oranges, and yellow fruit.

- vitamin B Complex is the name given to a group of around ten different B vitamins. Generally they can be found in whole grains, yeast, some leafy vegetables, and beans.

- vitamin C can be found in fresh fruits and vegetables.

- vitamin D can be found in fish liver oils and is also produced by the body through exposure to sunlight.

- Vitamin E is found in fresh vegetable oils, nuts, and fresh wheat germ.